Expert Techniques in Spine Surgery

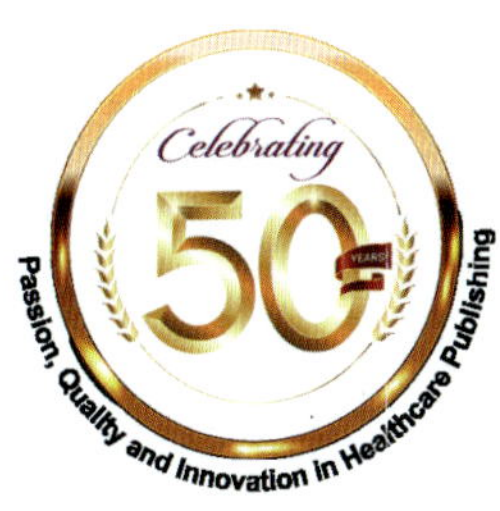

Expert Techniques in Spine Surgery

Editors

Alexander R Vaccaro MD PhD MBA
Richard H Rothman Professor and Chairman, Department of Orthopedic Surgery
Professor of Neurosurgery
Co-Director, Delaware Valley Spinal Cord Injury Center
Co-Chief of Spine Surgery
Sidney Kimmel Medical Center at Thomas Jefferson University
President, Rothman Institute
Philadelphia, Pennsylvania, USA

Arjun Sebastian MD MS
Assistant Professor of Orthopedic Surgery
Assistant Professor of Neurosurgery
Senior Associate Consultant
Mayo Clinic
Rochester, Minnesota, USA

Foreword

Michael Y Wang

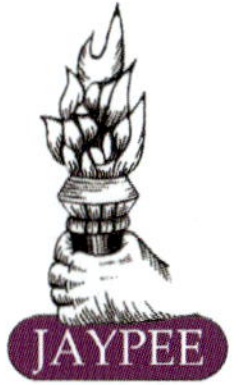

JAYPEE BROTHERS MEDICAL PUBLISHERS
The Health Sciences Publisher
New Delhi | London | Panama

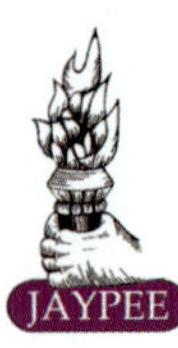

Jaypee Brothers Medical Publishers (P) Ltd

Headquarters

Jaypee Brothers Medical Publishers (P) Ltd
4838/24, Ansari Road, Daryaganj
New Delhi 110 002, India
Phone: +91-11-43574357
Fax: +91-11-43574314
E-mail: jaypee@jaypeebrothers.com

Overseas Offices

JP Medical Ltd
83 Victoria Street, London
SW1H 0HW (UK)
Phone: +44 20 3170 8910
Fax: +44 (0)20 3008 6180
E-mail: info@jpmedpub.com

Jaypee-Highlights Medical Publishers Inc
City of Knowledge, Bld. 235, 2nd Floor
Clayton, Panama City, Panama
Phone: +1 507-301-0496
Fax: +1 507-301-0499
E-mail: cservice@jphmedical.com

Jaypee Brothers Medical Publishers (P) Ltd
Bhotahity, Kathmandu, Nepal
Phone: +977-9741283608
E-mail: kathmandu@jaypeebrothers.com

Website: www.jaypeebrothers.com
Website: www.jaypeedigital.com

Inquiries for bulk sales may be solicited at: jaypee@jaypeebrothers.com

Expert Techniques in Spine Surgery

First Edition: **2020**

ISBN 978-93-5270-980-9

Printed at Replika Press Pvt. Ltd.

Dedicated to

This book to a very special person
Benjamin Francis Cottone, who aspires to one day be an orthopedic surgeon.
Ben, I am so impressed with your determination, skill, and thirst for knowledge.
These attributes paired with your affectionate personality will lead you to a thriving and successful future. I will be there to support you on your journey every step of the way.

Alexander R Vaccaro

Contributors

Alan Hilibrand

Alexander M Satin

Alexander R Vaccaro

Alexander Satin

Alfred J Pisano

Andrew Wright

A Noelle Larson

Arjun Sebastian

Chris Daniels

Christopher Kepler

Daniel N Kiridly

David A Essig

David Kaye

Dennis P Kurian

D Greg Anderson

Hannah Kirby

Jacob Borck

James McKenzie

Jeff S Silber

Kyle Nappo

Larry Lenke

Mark Kurd

Mohamad Bydon

Mohammed Ali Alvi

Nelson Saldua

Panagiotis Kerezoudis

Patrick Morrissey

Scott C Wagner

Tyler Kreitz

Foreword

The nature of modern spinal surgery is that it is a technically demanding subspecialty. This is coupled with the recent renaissance in methods for decompressing neural elements, reconstructing the spinal column, and achieving alignment goals, making this a challenging but dynamic field. Thus, practitioners of the art are seeking information about the most contemporary techniques.

It is in this context that *Expert Techniques in Spine Surgery* emerges. The document is edited by one of the most authoritative modern spine surgeons, Alexander R Vaccaro and an up and coing star Arjun Sebastian. Understanding that spinal surgeons are extremely busy, this book offers critical information delivered in a concise format. The topics covered are the most essential techniques employed in our field, and taken as a whole, the methods comprise roughly 80% of all spinal surgery as it is practiced in the United States. Thus, for the trainee who is stressed for time, this book is a fantastic quick and ready reference; for the busy practicing surgeon this book serves as a great refresher.

The organization of the chapters is systematic, covering the most essential aspects of the surgical intervention. In this manner, one is not muddled in a sea of details on the details on history, physiology, or irrelevant anatomy. Rather, the focus is on perfect surgical technique and its execution. Tips and pearls, case examples, and short video clips are offered to allow the reader to quickly focus on what often matters most: the intervention transpiring in the operating room.

In our current era where the sheer volume of information is often itself the problem, *Expert Techniques in Spine Surgery* is a welcome addition that achieves relevance through focus. I would recommend this book to practitioners at all levels who wish to refine their surgical abilities.

Michael Y Wang MD
Miami, Florida, USA

Preface

Spine surgery is a rapidly evolving field, with numerous advancements constantly being made to improve the overall safety and efficacy of various surgical procedures. With a greater understanding of spinal pathophysiology comes an array of modern surgical techniques that have been developed to allow surgeons to more precisely address specific pathoanatomy to improve a patient's quality of life. As the number of spine procedures continues to increase, it becomes increasingly important for surgeons to master more advanced techniques to provide patients with better long-term outcomes.

The editors of *"Expert Techniques in Spine Surgery"* have sought out the most frequently performed and most recently developed and refined procedures in spinal care to highlight in this book. A tireless effort has been put forth by the editors and authors to provide the reader with an easy to understand instructional treatise on open and minimally invasive methods to decompress, stabilize, and provide motion to the diseased spine.

"Expert Techniques in Spine Surgery" consists of 12 well-selected chapters, covering essential techniques in cervical, thoracic, and lumbar spine surgery with an emphasis on skillful surgical techniques and considerations. Each chapter follows a reproducible format with (1) an in-depth review of the relevant anatomy; (2) a thorough discourse of specific indications and contraindications for the procedure; (3) a methodical instructional guide for how to master the technique with a variety of special caveats that only the most experienced surgeons are aware of; (4) the most up-to-date discussion of outcomes that validate the use of these contemporary techniques; (5) an extensive guide to potential complications that may arise intraoperatively and perioperatively; (6) a well-crafted case presentation to tie concepts together; and (7) a variety of detailed imaging and illustrations to visually guide readers through the complexities of each technique.

This anthology of complex spinal techniques has been carefully crafted as a teaching tool for medical students, orthopedic residents, spine fellows, and young spine attendings, in a collective effort to improve the administration of complex spine care to patients around the world. We are confident that this textbook will serve as a benchmark of quality spine care and a proper reference guide for leaders in this exciting and innovative field.

Alexander R Vaccaro
Arjun Sebastian

Acknowledgments

I would like to acknowledge the incredible hard work that my co-editor Arjun Sebastian has put into making this book a reality. Often an editor needs to completely rewrite chapters or write an absent chapter never submitted. Arjun has taken on that role and has done a spectacular job. Additionally, I would like to thank the research staff at the Rothman Institute, Philadelphia, Pennsylvania, USA, for their support throughout the year in assisting in all aspects of scientific inquiry supporting the fellows and surgical staff. My hat is off to the leader of this group Dhruv Goyal for his loyalty and commitment to this academic mission.

I am thankful to Shri Jitendar P Vij (Group Chairman), Mr Ankit Vij (Managing Director), Mr MS Mani (Group President), Ms Chetna Malhotra Vohra (Associate Director—Content Strategy), Ms Pooja Bhandari (Production Head) and Ms Prerna Bajaj (Development Editor) of M/s Jaypee Brothers Medical Publishers (P) Ltd, New Delhi, India, for giving a go-ahead at the very beginning and helping us in every way possible to bring out this book.

Alexander R Vaccaro

Contents

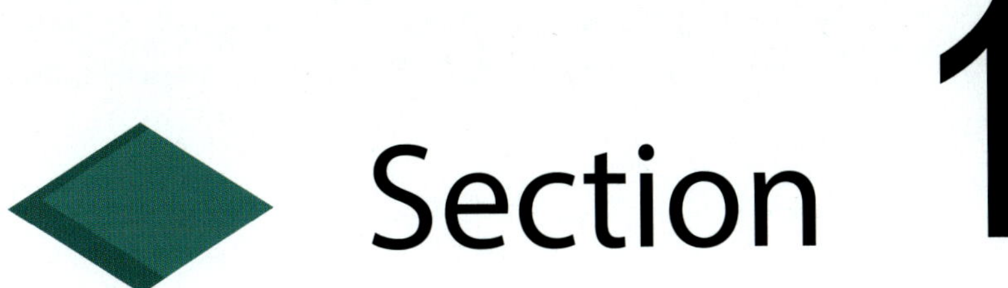

Section 1

Cervical

- Posterior Cervical Foraminotomy
- Cervical Corpectomy
- Cervical Total Disc Arthroplasty
- Cervical Laminoplasty

CHAPTER

1

Posterior Cervical Foraminotomy

Alfred J Pisano, Scott C Wagner

ANATOMY

Nerves

At each cervical level, a pair of ventral and dorsal roots exits the spinal cord. The dorsal roots unite with the dorsal root ganglion, which is found within the neural foramen. Just distal to this point, the ventral and dorsal roots coalesce to form a spinal nerve. Each spinal nerve runs obliquely out of the neural foramen and immediately branches into anterior and posterior rami. The posterior rami supply the paraspinal musculature, and the anterior rami supply the remainder of the body. As compared to the thoracic and lumbar nerves, cervical nerves are more transversely oriented.

Within the neural foramen, each cervical nerve is bordered anteriorly by the cervical disc corresponding to its level and posteriorly by the superior articular processes of the caudal vertebra. Cephalad and caudal pedicles border the cervical nerves superiorly and inferiorly. The anterior rami course ventrally in a groove along the transverse process. The nerve is directly dorsal to the vertebral artery and the vein in the transverse process (Fig. 1.1).

Osteology

The cervical vertebrae have unique articulations. The cervical spine is composed of an uncovertebral joint and two facet joints, which form a tripod. The articulations of vertebral bodies form uncovertebral joints. In the coronal plane, each superior endplate is concave and forms two uncinate processes laterally. Each uncinate process articulates with a convex inferior endplate of the adjacent vertebral body to form an uncovertebral joint.

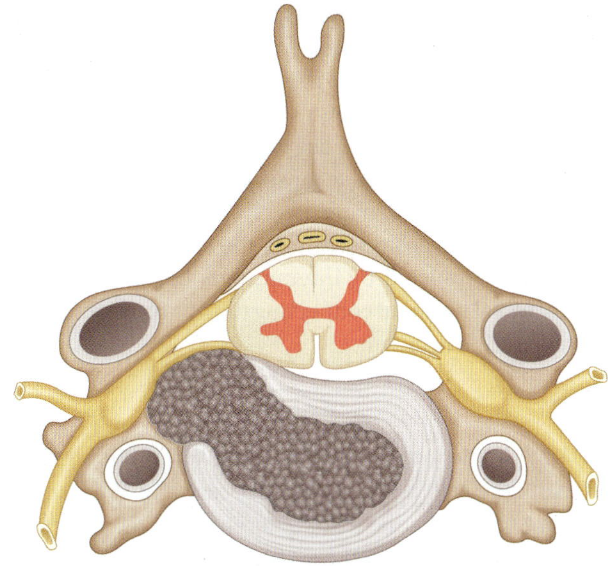

Fig. 1.1: A cross-sectional anatomy of a cervical disc herniation. Recognizing the orientation of disc relative to the pedicle is the key to performing the procedure.
Source: Simeone FA. (2016). Surgery for Cervical Radicular Pain. [online] Available from https://musculoskeletalkey.com/surgery-for-cervical-radicular-pain/ [Accessed November 2018].

Superior and inferior articular processes form facet joints, which are oriented in the coronal plane. The articular processes are stout columns of bone that form the lateral masses of the subaxial spine.[1] Superior articular processes (SAPs) project superiorly from the pedicle and face posteriorly, while inferior articular processes project inferiorly from the pedicle and face anteriorly. The SAP is closest in relation to the cervical nerve, as it forms the dorsal surface of the neural foramen.

Pedicles project posterolaterally from the vertebral body, and are oriented approximately 90° in the transverse plane and 75° in the sagittal plane.[2] The pedicles exit the vertebral body approximately midway between the superior and inferior endplates so that the superior and inferior vertebral notches are similar in dimension. The apposition of these notches creates the neural foramen. Each cervical nerve passes cephalad to its corresponding pedicle and sits on the floor of the neural foramen in direct contact with the superior cortex of the pedicle.[3]

Transverse processes are formed by anterior and posterior roots in the cervical spine. Anterior roots project laterally from the vertebral body, and posterior roots project laterally from the pedicle. These roots join to form transverse foramina, through which vertebral arteries and veins pass through. Each transverse process also has a groove on its cephalad surface, which carries the cervical nerve from the neural foramen. Laterally, the transverse process is bifid and forms an anterior and posterior tubercle. The anterior and posterior cervical muscles insert on each tubercle.

The laminae form the dorsal covering of the spinal cord. The laminae are shingled such that each cephalad lamina overlays a caudal lamina. The ligamentum flavum connects adjacent lamina by originating from the superior aspect of the caudal laminae and inserting approximately one-third up on the undersurface of the cephalad laminae. The ligaments are separated by a small space midline and extend laterally to the facet capsule. The interlaminar space is wider in the cervical spine than in the lumbar spine, which is important to note for surgical approach. Immediately deep to the ligamentum flavum is the dura mater.

Spinous processes project posteriorly from the confluence of laminae. Adjacent spinous processes are connected by interspinous ligaments. The supraspinous ligament is the most dorsal ligament connecting the tips of the spinous processes and is confluent with the nuchal ligament.

Vasculature

The vertebral arteries branch off the subclavian arteries and enter the transverse foramen of the sixth cervical vertebrae in most cases. In the transverse foramen, vertebral arteries are ventral to the exiting cervical nerves. Transverse processes protect the vertebral arteries as long as the vertebral artery does not take an anomalous course and the transverse process is not compromised by pathologic processes or congenital anomalies. One large study demonstrated anomalous vertebral arteries occur in up to 7% of patients.[4]

Musculature

The musculature of the posterior neck is divided into three layers. The trapezius comprises the superficial layer. The splenius capitis comprises the intermediate layer. The deep layer includes the semispinalis capitis, semispinalis cervicis, and multifidus. These muscles are generally not identified intraoperatively, as the surgical approach for posterior cervical foraminotomy (PCF) dissects these muscles subperiosteally from the spinous processes.

INDICATIONS

A PCF is indicated for the treatment of cervical radiculopathy. In order to be eligible for a PCF, patients should experience symptoms of radicular pain, weakness, with or without numbness. These symptoms should be corroborated by a physical examination and advanced imaging demonstrating a focal neurologic compression corresponding to the affected nerve root.

It is essential to understand the natural history of cervical radiculopathy to avoid overtreatment. In their classic study, Lees and Turner[5] evaluated the natural history of cervical radiculopathy in 41 patients with a follow-up of up to 10 years. They found that 45% of patients had a single episode of symptoms, 30% had intermittent symptoms, and 25% had persistent symptoms.[5] A systematic review demonstrated similar findings: a significant proportion of patients experienced clinical improvement within 4–6 months after the onset of symptoms. Additionally, approximately 80% of patients had a complete recovery in 24–36 months.[6]

A trial of nonoperative management should be considered prior to surgical intervention. Patients should be initially managed with conservative measures and educated about the natural history of the disease. A first-line treatment options include nonsteroidal anti-inflammatory drugs (NSAIDs), physical therapy, and activity modification. Selective nerve root injections (SNRIs) are available as a second-line intervention. SNRIs have both diagnostic and therapeutic efficacy. If an SNRI provides relief, it is reasonable to expect a similar and prolonged result with PCF.

Posterior cervical foraminotomy directly decompresses the cervical nerve in the lateral canal and neural foramen. Therefore, PCF can technically be performed to address any focal pathology occurring in these areas. A lateral soft disc herniation at a single level is the ideal indication for PCF. However, PCF also has utility in several other clinical scenarios.

Posterior cervical foraminotomy is generally more effective at treating soft discs than hard discs. It is also better suited for addressing focal pathology rather than a diffuse process. Soft discs typically represent focal neurologic compression. Conversely, hard discs typically represent a more diffuse degenerative process. Soft discs can be directly decompressed from a posterior approach, while hard discs are technically more difficult to decompress from a posterior approach. A posterior decompression of hard discs may necessitate excessive nerve retraction causing iatrogenic injury. Therefore, a patient with a symptomatic isolated soft disc herniation is an ideal candidate for PCF.

Occasionally, disc herniations occur at multiple levels or bilaterally. In these cases, a multilevel PCF may be indicated. It is important to differentiate multilevel herniations from diffuse spondylotic disease, as the latter may be better treated with anterior or combined approaches. The concern with multilevel and bilateral PCF is the potential for destabilization of the spine. Biomechanical studies demonstrate that retaining 50% of each facet may prevent instability of the spine.[7] An excessive decompression risks iatrogenic spondylolisthesis, which may require fusion.

Finally, PCF is a useful technique for patients who are poor candidates for an anterior approach or for those who are at risk of developing a pseudarthrosis. Patients who have undergone previous anterior approaches have increased risk with another anterior approach. If the pathology can be managed from a posterior approach, PCF may be a viable alternative to revision anterior decompression. Similarly, patients who are at risk of developing a pseudarthrosis may be considered for PCF rather than anterior cervical discectomy and fusion (ACDF).

The absolute contraindication to PCF is cervical myelopathy, as PCF will not adequately decompress central cord compression.

TECHNIQUE

Preoperative Planning

A careful interpretation of imaging is essential to the success of PCF. Generally, a magnetic resonance imaging (MRI) is used to localize and characterize the pathology. The areas of compression must be identified preoperatively in order to adequately address them intraoperatively. Compression may be due to anterior structures, such as protruded disc or osteophytes. Compression may also occur from posterior structures, such as hypertrophied ligamentum flavum. Depending on the area of compression, the nerve root may need to be retracted to adequately decompress the foramen. It is also important to note the consistency of the tissue causing the compression. Soft discs may be easier to decompress without nerve root retraction, whereas hard discs may necessitate direct visualization and more aggressive nerve root retraction.

Equipment

A fluoroscope or plain X-ray and a spinal needle or other markers are necessary for localization. A high-speed side-cutting burr is used for the majority of the decompression. It is also important to have 1 and 2 mm Kerrison rongeurs available for foraminal decompression. A nerve root retractor and probe are needed to manipulate the nerve root and evaluate the extent of decompression. Hemostatic agents are useful for visualization.

Positioning

The patient is placed in the prone position on a Jackson frame table with bivector Gardner-Wells tong traction (Orthopaedic Systems, Inc., Union City, CA). Bivector traction allows for easy transition from flexion to extension as necessary. Bolsters are placed under the clavicles to allow for flexion of the head. The patient's neck is in slight flexion, as this unshingles the facets, allows for better exposure, and minimizes the need for extensive resection of the inferior articular process (IAP). The patient is also placed in slight reverse Trendelenburg to reduce venous bleeding and cerebrospinal fluid (CSF) pressure. The shoulders are taped down when approaching lower cervical levels to allow for better radiographic exposure. The chest and the abdomen are supported on bolsters, which allows the abdomen to hang free. The legs are supported in a sling and flexed at the knee with pillows (Fig. 1.2).

Approach

One approach is to make a midline incision centered over the spinous process of the cephalad level involved. A spinal needle is used to localize the level radiographically. The skin is incised sharply and then electrocautery is used to dissect midline through the ligamentum nuchae to the level of the spinous process. At this point, the periosteum is released off the side of the spinous process of the involved side. This subperiosteal dissection is performed with a Cobb elevator, and the dissection

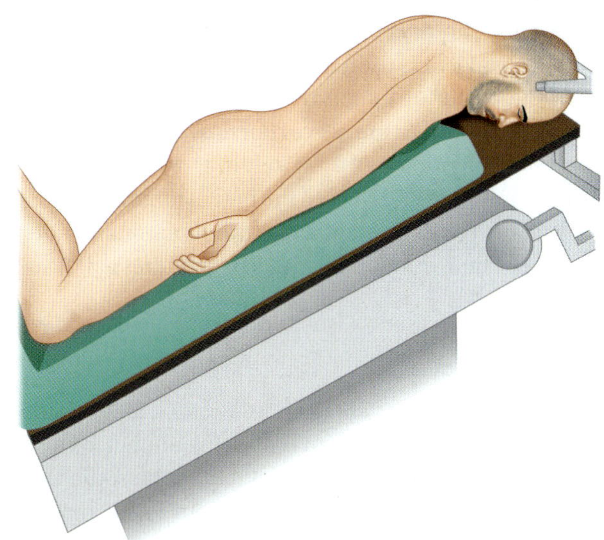

Fig. 1.2: Patient should be positioned utilizing cranial tongs and reverse Trendelenburg to minimize epidural bleeding.
Source: Simeone FA. (2016). Surgery for Cervical Radicular Pain. [online] Available from https://musculoskeletalkey.com/surgery-for-cervical-radicular-pain/ [Accessed November 2018].

is brought down over the lamina. It is important to ensure that the instrument does not penetrate the interlaminar space, which is wider in the cervical spine than in the lumbar spine. The subperiosteal dissection is continued laterally over the lateral mass and the facet joint. Do not violate the facet capsule, as this can lead to facet arthrosis or instability.[8]

An alternative minimally invasive approach may also be utilized. In this approach, the targeted facet joint is targeted fluoroscopically. A 2 cm incision is made off midline and serial dilation is performed with a tubular retractor system. Care is taken to identify the lamina and facet joint. The operation then proceeds in a similar fashion to the open approach.

Decompression

Once the lamina and facet joint of the desired level are exposed, the decompression is performed. A high-speed 2 mm acorn-shaped carbide tip cutting burr is used to resect the inferior half of the cephalad lamina. The superior third of the caudal lamina is also resected. The decompression is then carried out laterally to the facet joint. The medial third to one half of the facet joint is removed as necessary. Removing more than 50% of the facet may lead to iatrogenic instability.[7] The ligamentum flavum is then removed with a 1 or 2 mm Kerrison rongeur. At this point, the nerve root is visualized and bony resection is complete.

The nerve root is then decompressed on all sides. The herniated disc is generally found anterior and caudal to the nerve root. The nerve root is therefore retracted superiorly, and a nerve hook is swept anterior to the nerve root to release any fragments. A pituitary rongeur is used to remove any visible fragments. If an incision must be made in the posterior longitudinal ligament (PLL), the knife is directed inferiorly and laterally parallel to the nerve root to avoid nerve injury. The nerve root should not be retracted inferiorly, as this is likely to cause an iatrogenic neuropraxia. A probe is then used to follow the nerve into the neural foramen (Figs. 1.3 and 1.4). The SAP is dorsal, the disc is ventral, and pedicles are superior and inferior to the nerve root. Each of these structures must be adequately addressed based on presenting pathology.

Closure

Prior to closure, it is essential to achieve hemostasis. Failure to do so can lead to nerve root or cord compression. Gelfoam is a useful adjunct for hemostasis. A drain is generally not utilized after PCF. Fascia is sutured to the supraspinous ligament in watertight fashion followed by closure of subcutaneous and cutaneous layers.

Postoperative Protocol

Generally, PCF is performed at the same day of surgery. Given that there is no need for fusion, motion is not limited postoperatively. A soft collar may be used to relieve pain.

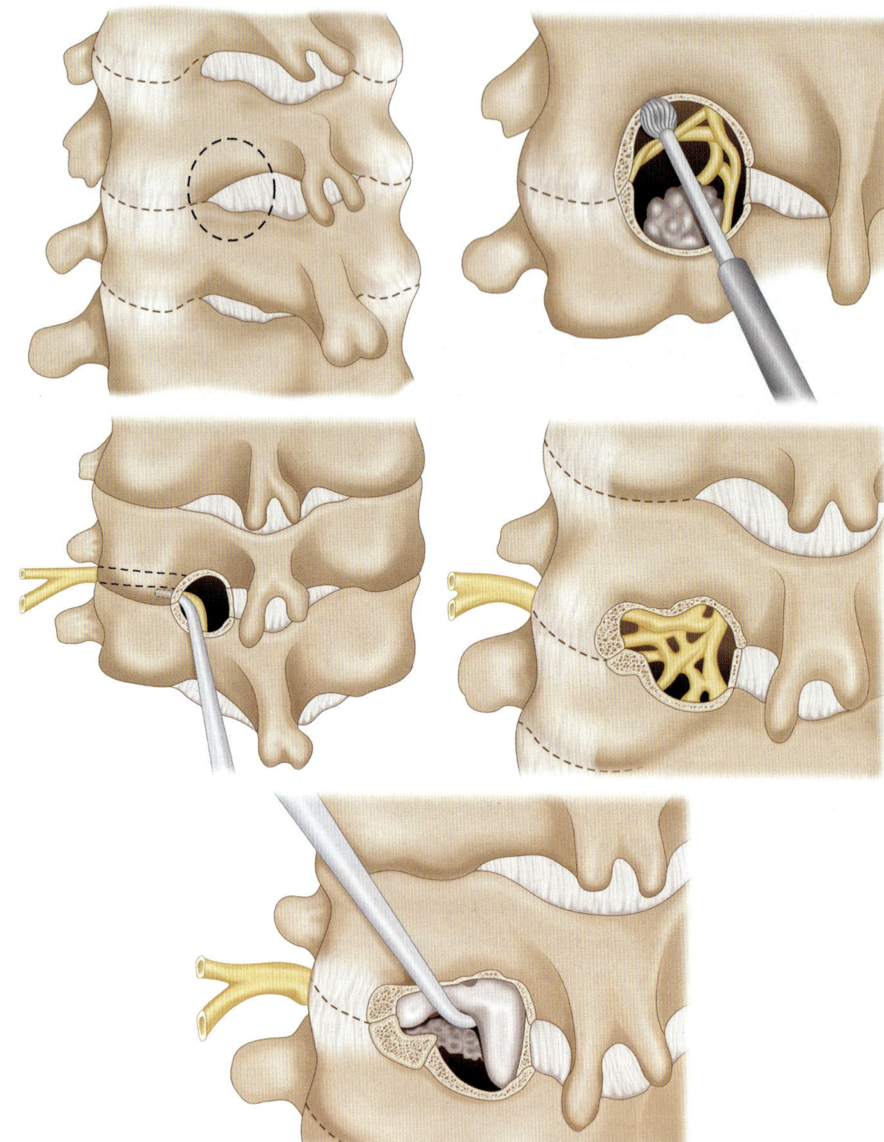

Fig. 1.3: Access for the foraminotomy requires identification of the V-shaped intersection of the cranial and caudal lamina with the medial aspect of the facet joint. Following laminotomy, the course of the nerve should be delineated by palpating pedicle utilizing a nerve hooking. Decompression proceeds with the foraminotomy taking care to not overresect the facet joint. Following this, the vascular plexus overlying the nerve root and disc may be identified and cauterized as needed. The nerve root can then be gently retracted cranially to access disk fragments.
Source: Simeone FA. (2016). Surgery for Cervical Radicular Pain. [online] Available from https://musculoskeletalkey.com/surgery-for-cervical-radicular-pain/ [Accessed November 2018].

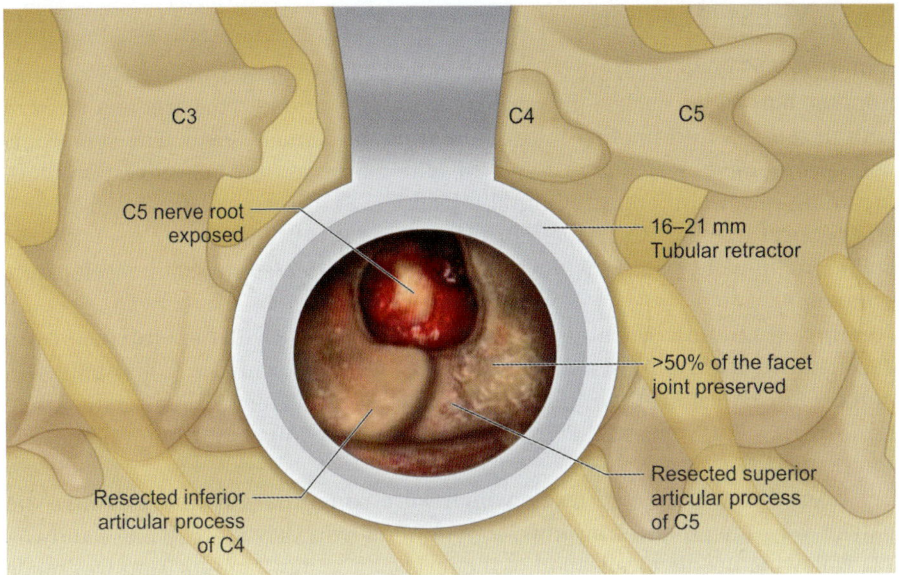

Fig. 1.4: Example of the exposure needed to perform a posterior cervical foraminotomy through a tubular minimally invasive approach. Again it is the key to avoid overresection of the facet joint. *Source:* J Spinal Disord Tech. 2015 Oct;28(8):295-7. doi: 10.1097/BSD.0000000000000318.

PEARLS

- The position of the patient is in slight reverse Trendelenburg to improve visualization.
- Flex the neck slightly to unshingle the laminae during decompression.
- Use 1 and 2 mm Kerrison rongeurs to perform foraminal decompression.
- Retract the nerve cranially, and use probe to sweep out herniated disc material.
- Confirm adequate decompression by probing the neural foramen.

PITFALLS

- Do not strip facet capsule during approach, as this may lead to instability.
- Do not resect greater than 50% of facet, as this may also lead to instability.
- If an incision must be made into the PLL, ensure the knife is directed caudally and laterally, paralleling the nerve root to prevent iatrogenic injury.
- Ensure adequate hemostasis prior to closure.

OUTCOMES

Multiple studies have demonstrated the efficacy of PCF in treating cervical radiculopathy. In a well-indicated patient, PCF is highly effective with minimal risks. In a large case series of 846 posterior laminoforaminotomies with an average follow-up of 2.8 years, Henderson et al.[9] found that patients had a 96% rate of relief of significant arm pain and/or paresthesias. Additionally, a 98% rate of motor deficit resolution was observed, and 91% of patients described themselves as "good or excellent" postoperatively.[9] Similarly, a case series with longer follow-up of 6 years demonstrated that 95% of patients achieved excellent outcomes.[10] A large series of patients treated on an outpatient basis demonstrated a 93% rate of good or excellent outcomes.[11] This study demonstrates that the PCF can be performed on an outpatient basis because it is safe and well tolerated.

Although it is clear that PCF is an effective treatment of cervical radiculopathy, few studies have evaluated the efficacy of PCF as compared to ACDF. A systematic review identified one low quality study comparing clinical outcomes between PCF, ACDF, and anterior cervical discectomy (ACD) in the treatment of acute cervical disc herniation. At 2 months, pain relief, resolution of neurologic deficits, and return to work was equivalent between all three groups. ACDF and PCF had equivalent reoperation rates, but reoperations were most common in adjacent levels in the ACDF group and at the index level in the PCF group.[12,13] A prospective study demonstrated conflicting results. In a comparison of anterior and posterior decompressions for posterolateral soft disc herniations, ACDF patients fared significantly better with a 94% rate of excellent or good outcomes compared to 75% in the PCF group.[14]

COMPLICATIONS

Posterior cervical foraminotomy has a low risk of complications. The most commonly reported complication in a case series by Williams[15] was a transiently worsened cervical radiculopathy or paresis, which was identified in 8% of patients. However, these symptoms resolved in less than 6 days in a vast majority of patients.[15]

Air embolism is a rare but potentially dangerous complication associated with PCF. Zeidman and Ducker[16] reported a 2% rate of air embolism in patients who underwent PCF. All events occurred in patients who were in the sitting position when PCF was performed. The authors do not comment on the clinical effects of the emboli. Alternatively, a large case series by Henderson et al.[9] demonstrated no air emboli in over 800 cases performed in the sitting position. We advocate reverse Trendelenburg positioning, which mitigates the risk of air embolism while also improving the surgical field visualization.

Postoperative segmental instability is another common complication after PCF. Bony resection and facet capsule resection both play a role in postoperative instability. In a cadaveric model, Zdeblick et al.[7] demonstrated that greater than 50% facet resection led to a significant decrease in torsional and translational stiffness. Similarly, facet capsule resection also led to an increase in instability. Greater than 50% capsule resection led to a statistically significant increase in segmental motion in flexion.[8] Clinical data correlating the amount of resection to rates of postoperative instability is limited. However, a good rule of thumb is to resect less than half of the facet and its capsule.

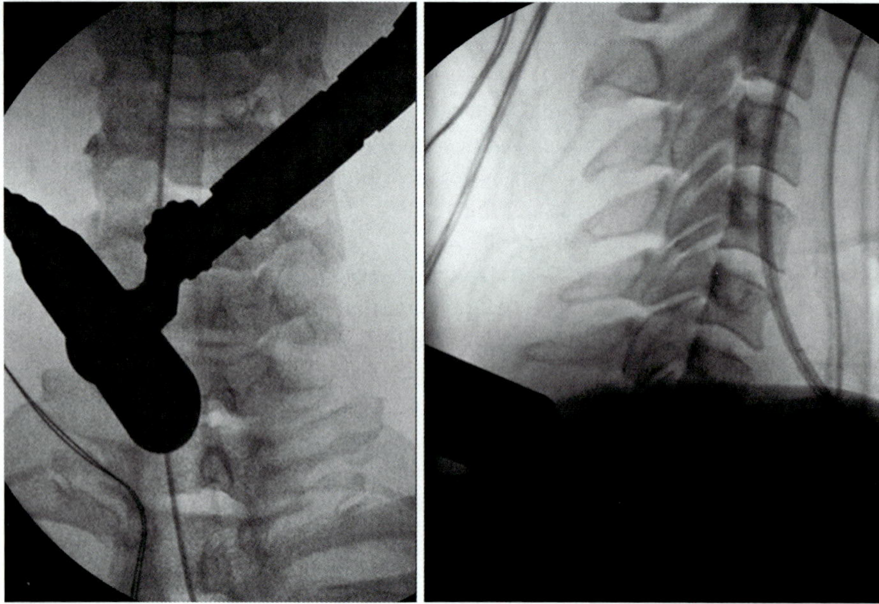

Fig. 1.5: Following needle localization, the tube is docked at the C7-T1 facet joint. Often caudal levels are difficult to image on a lateral image, for that reason, an AP fluoroscope image taken orthogonal to the disc space can ensure proper tube positioning (AP: anteroposterior).

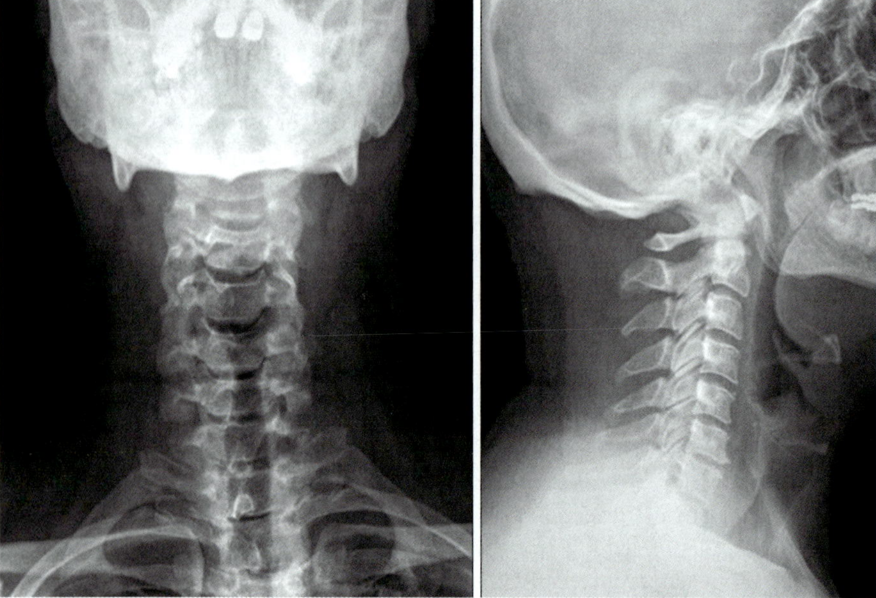

Fig. 1.6: At final follow-up at 3 months, radiographic imaging demonstrates minimal bony resection and no evidence of instability.

CASE PRESENTATION

A 48-year-old male presented with severe left arm radicular pain. Pain radiates from the base of his neck to the periscapular region and into the arm and forearm with numbness and tingling in the long, ring, and small finger. The symptoms were progressive over the past year despite extensive nonoperative treatment including physical therapy, epidural injections, anti-inflammatory medications, and cervical traction. The patient has increasing loss of function in his left hand and more difficulty with activities of daily living. He denies any frank myelopathic symptoms.

On radiographic imaging, he is found to have cervical spondylosis with degenerative changes most notable at the C6-7 level. No evidence of instability was noted. On cervical MRI, he was noted to have severe left-sided neural foraminal stenosis at C6-7 as well as C7-T1. No evidence of cord compression or myelomalacia was noted.

Given the two affected levels which were concordant with symptoms, the patient was offered and consented to a minimally invasive PCF at C6-7 and C7-T1. Following needle localization of the levels, a roughly 2 cm incision was made in line with the facet joints. Serial dilation was performed taking care to verify the correct levels on both anteroposterior (AP) and lateral fluoroscopic images (Fig. 1.5). Following tube docking, cautery was used to identify the lamina and the facet joint. A high-speed burr was utilized to make a laminotomy and thin the bone over the medial aspect of the facet joint. This was then resected with a right angle curette and Kerrison rongeurs. After achieving hemostasis, a nerve hook was utilized to verify decompression and probe for disc fragments.

At 3-month follow-up, the patient was doing well with complete resolution of the left arm pain. Radiographs did not demonstrate any evidence of instability and the patient was allowed to return to all normal activities (Fig. 1.6).

REFERENCES

1. Schwender JD, Foley KT, Longston TH, et al. Rothman - Simeone: The Spine; 2006. doi:10.1016/B978-1-4160-6726-9.00012-2.
2. Ebraheim NA, Xu R, Knight T, et al. Morphometric evaluation of lower cervical pedicle and its projection. Spine (Phila Pa 1976). 1997;22(1):1-6.
3. Xu R, Kang A, Ebraheim N, et al. Neural foramen relationship. Spine (Phila Pa 1976). 1999;24(5):451-4.
4. Uchino A, Saito N, Takahashi M, et al. Variations in the origin of the vertebral artery and its level of entry into the transverse foramen diagnosed by CT angiography. Neuroradiol. 2013;55(5):585-94.
5. Lees F, Turner A. Natural history and prognosis of cervical spondylosis. Br Med J. 1963;2(5373):1607-10.
6. Wong JJ, Fccs C, Pierre C, et al. The course and prognostic factors of symptomatic cervical disc herniation with radiculopathy: a systematic review of the literature. Spine J. 2014;14:1781-9.

7. Zdeblick TA, Mccabe R, Zou D, et al. Cervical stability after foraminotomy. JBJS. 1992;74A(1):22-7.
8. Zdeblick TA, Abitbol JJ, Kunz DN, et al. Cervical stability after sequential capsule resection. Spine (Phila Pa 1976). 1993;18(14):2005-8.
9. Henderson C, Hennessy R, Shuey H, et al. Posterior-lateral foraminotomy as an exclusive operative technique for cervical radiculopathy: a review of 846 consecutively operated cases. Neurosurgery. 1983;13(5):504-12.
10. Silveri CP, Simpson JM, Simeone FA, et al. Cervical disk disease and the keyhole foraminotomy: Proven efficacy at extended long-term follow up. Orthopedics. 1997;20(8):687-92.
11. Tomaras CR, Blacklock JB, Parker WD, et al. Outpatient surgical treatment of cervical radiculopathy. J Neurosurg. 1997;87(1):41-3.
12. Gebremariam L, Koes BW, Peul WC, et al. Evaluation of treatment effectiveness for the herniated cervical disc. Spine (Phila Pa 1976). 2012;37(2):E109-18.
13. Wirth FP, Dowd GC, Sanders HF, et al. Cervical discectomy. A prospective analysis of three operative techniques. Surg Neurol. 2000;53(4):340-6.
14. Herkowitz HN, Kurz LT, Overholt DP. Surgical management of cervical soft disc herniation. A comparison between the anterior and posterior approach. Spine (Phila Pa 1976). 1990;15(10):1026-30.
15. Williams RW. Microcervical foraminotomy. Spine (Phila Pa 1976). 1983;8(7): 708-16.
16. Zeidman SM, Ducker TB. Posterior cervical laminoforaminotomy for radiculopathy review of 172 cases. Neurosurgery. 1993;33(3):356-62.

CHAPTER

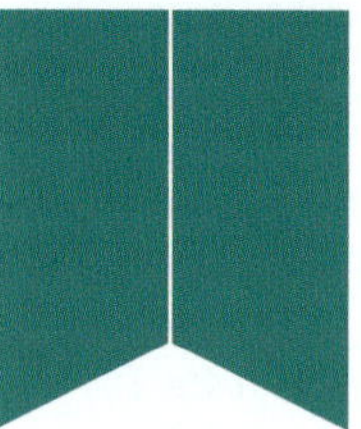

2

Cervical Corpectomy

James McKenzie, Arjun Sebastian, Christopher Kepler

ANATOMY

Upper and Subaxial Cervical Spine Overview

The cervical spine contains seven vertebral segments and eight nerve roots whose function provides motor and sensory innervation to the bilateral upper extremities. Along with innervation, the cervical spine enables neck flexion, extension, rotation, and lateral bending. The normal sagittal alignment ranges from 20° to 40° of lordosis. It is typically subdivided into two parts—(1) the upper and (2) subaxial cervical spine. The upper cervical spine consists of the first two cervical vertebrae, the atlas and axis, respectively. The atlas is a uniquely-shaped ring structure which connects the occiput to the rest of the cervical spine and is responsible for about 50% of the neck flexion and extension. The foramen magnum provides a large conduit for the traversing spinal cord which enlarges in the cephalad direction toward the central nervous system. The atlas also articulates with the conforming axis via the odontoid process and is responsible for approximately 60% of the neck rotation.[1] The flexibility and durability of the upper cervical spine is augmented by a complex of ligaments surrounding the atlanto-dens articulation with the transverse ligament preventing anterior atlas translation and apical and alar ligaments limiting excessive neck rotation.[2,3]

The subaxial cervical spine includes the third to the seventh cervical vertebrae with repetitive osteology and articulations which provides the remainder of neck flexion, extension, rotation, and lateral bending in equal amounts. In the axial plane, each vertebra surrounds the neural foramen posteriorly with the spinous process and lamina which connects to the pedicle and vertebral body anteriorly. Laterally, the transverse foramina protect both the vertebral arteries. In the coronal plane, the zygapophyseal joints include the superior and inferior articular facets joining each cervical vertebra to its adjacent level in a posteromedial to posterolateral orientation in the caudal direction.[4] In the sagittal plane, the neural foramina lies anteromedial to the transverse foramina and is the outlet for the spinal nerve roots which then divides into the ventral motor branch and dorsal sensory branch. The entire cervical spine is invested by the anterior longitudinal ligament (ALL) and posterior longitudinal ligament (PLL). The ALL lies just anterior to the cervical bodies and runs distally into the thoracolumbar spine. The PLL lies within the spinal canal directly on the posterior aspect of the vertebral bodies and similarly continues inferiorly through the rest of the vertebral column. Between each vertebral body lies the cervical disc which functions as a shock-absorber to the axial load of the cranium and allows space for the surrounding neurovascular structures.[5]

Surface Anatomy and Landmarks

The surface anatomy of the anterior neck provides reliable approximations of cervical vertebral levels with simple palpation on physical examination. Given the numerous critical structures superficial to the anterior cervical spine, it is vital for the surgeon to understand the surface anatomy prior to dissection. Such estimates assist in the appropriate incision placement for adequate surgical exposure. Furthermore, these landmarks are fairly reproducible regardless of patient age, body mass index (BMI), or relative neck habitus.[6]

Starting cephalad, the hard palate of the mouth corresponds with the anterior arch of the atlas. The lower border of the mandible correlates with C2-3. The physician can further elucidate the C3 level by palpating the lateral aspects of the C-shaped hyoid bone which rests posteromedial to the inferior edge of the mandible. Anterior to the C4 level, lies the superior aspect of the thyroid cartilage, which then can be traced inferiorly to the cricothyroid ligament which is an avascular structure critical to establishing an emergency airway. Just distal to this ligament is the cricoid cartilage which corresponds to the C6 level. Finally, the carotid tubercle, a structure just posteromedial to the distal aspect of the carotid artery and its pulse is the landmark for the C7 vertebral level. Inferiorly lies the suprasternal notch and the superior aspect of the manubrium, marking the transition into the ribs and thoracic spine posteriorly.[5]

Another important surface landmark is the sternocleidomastoid muscle (SCM). The SCM innervated by the spinal accessory nerve, originates at the mastoid process of the temporal bone of the cranium and travels obliquely across the neck, splitting into two muscle bellies where it inserts onto the medial clavicle and manubrium of the sternum, respectively.[7] The SCM particularly the posterior aspect can be the lateral border for the initial incision from the midline of the neck when planning the surgical approach. Fortunately, the SCM remains a palpable anatomic landmark for most patients regardless of body habitus or neck length.

INDICATIONS

Anterior cervical corpectomy and fusion (ACCF) involves the bony resection of the cervical vertebrae along with the superior and inferior vertebral discs which provide significant decompression of the spinal cord with limited manipulation. ACCF is typically indicated when anterior cervical discectomy and fusion (ACDF) would not allow sufficient decompression of the spinal cord. This is often the case with multilevel cervical spondylosis, ossification of the PLL (OPLL), mechanical failure of the cervical vertebrae due to metastatic lesions, osteomyelitis, severe trauma, or a congenitally stenotic spinal canal.[8] Patients suffering from these disease processes will present with direct spinal cord compression and myelopathic symptoms, which usually fail conservative treatment.

Preoperative assessment and proper patient selection is critical for the surgeon to determine the surgical technique necessary to provide a successful decompression and construct amenable to fusion. Proper imaging, including four radiographic views of the cervical spine with dynamic flexion and extension, magnetic resonance imaging (MRI) and possibly computed tomography (CT) scan are required and compared with the clinical presentation to determine the best surgical plan. Vertebral body deformities, compressive lesions extending posterior to the vertebral body, severe anterior osteophytes, and confluent stenosis from one vertebral disc to the adjacent one will often necessitate ACCF over ACDF.[9,10]

Correction of cervical malalignment is another important consideration for surgical planning. Patients with significant kyphotic deformity can have the spinal cord draped over the degenerative anterior osteophytes at multiple levels in the cervical spine. Correcting this alignment closer to normal anatomic lordosis demands substantial extension and distraction around compressed and inflamed neural elements. Such a correction lends itself to ACCF which allows the requisite space for the spinal cord and neural elements to realign and limit the risk of iatrogenic traction and damage to the neural elements.[11]

TECHNIQUE

Operative Instrumentation and Patient Monitoring

The instruments required for surgery include intraoperative imaging and surgical loupes for the surgeon and assistant to safely dissect during the approach. A sterile operating microscope may also be used which aids the surgeon in the precise resection of the vertebral body and PLL while limiting the risk of iatrogenic injury to the surrounding neurovascular structures such as the vertebral artery and the spinal cord. Intraoperative fluoroscopy or plain radiography is also utilized to assess hardware and screw placement following a corpectomy and graft placement. The removal of the vertebral body, osteophytes, and ligamentous structures requires Kerrison and pituitary rongeurs, cervical curettes, and a high-speed burr. External traction may be necessary during the cervical correction in which Gardner-Wells tongs are placed 1 cm cranial to the outer helix of the ear in line with the external auditory meatus with the patient's head placed in a Mayfield horseshoe to enable proper axially- oriented traction. Appropriate retraction devices within the surgical bed such as self-retractors assist in proper surgical exposure at various points in the case. Finally, an anterior plating system and grafting material such as iliac crest bone allograft or perioperatively-harvested autograft are necessary for the fusion construct following corpectomy and decompression.

Intraoperative neuromonitoring (ION) with somatosensory evoked potentials (SSEPs) and motor-evoked potentials (MEPs) are utilized by the authors to assess the possible perioperative iatrogenic spinal cord injury or ischemia. Especially in patients with significant preoperative myelopathy, baseline SSEPs and MEPs should be obtained prior to and following patient positioning to make sure that the anesthetized patient can safely tolerate the procedure. ION at regular intervals during the procedure provides a sensitive and specific determination of overall nerve function and has been found to be efficacious for ACCF which carries a higher risk of neurologic injury in comparison to ACDFs.[12]

Proper coordination with the anesthesia team is vital to the success and safety of the procedure. Unless contraindicated, patients with significant cord compression should receive an arterial line to allow precise monitoring and adjustment of the mean arterial pressure (MAP) during the case. Perioperative hypotension places the spinal cord at risk for ischemic injury so an MAP above 85 mm Hg in the setting of significant cord compression is recommended during ACCF. Preoperative evaluation of the cervical stability, particularly following spinal cord injury, is important to determine whether the patient's neck can be manipulated during the process of endotracheal intubation.

Consideration must be made as to the laterality of the surgical incision. The recurrent laryngeal nerve (RLN) is a structure that can cross the surgical field during the approach. Injury to the laryngeal nerve can cause voice hoarseness and dysphonia to the patient. The left RLN nerve for most patients reliably tracks between the trachea and the esophagus in the midline of the neck having come off of the vagus nerve at the arch of the aorta. The right RLN usually comes around the right subclavian artery and runs along the trachea tracking medially in the caudal portion of the cervical spine, anywhere from C6-T1.[13] Therefore, the authors recommend a left-sided anterior approach to the cervical spine if possible. If there is a history of revision surgery or prior injury to the RLN, evaluation of the vocal cords preoperatively by an otolaryngologist may be necessary to determine the appropriate laterality of the approach. If there is prior injury and/or dysfunction to the RLN on one side, that side will be utilized again to prevent complete RLN palsy.[5]

Patient Positioning

The patient is placed on a regular operating room table in a supine position. Once endotracheal intubation is complete and the airway secured, all neuromonitoring is placed at the appropriate locations and baseline SSEPs and MEPs are obtained. If necessary, the patient's head may gently be placed into the Mayfield horseshoe and the Gardner-Wells tongs are placed with gentle traction applied. The authors prefer 10 pounds of traction slowly placed in intervals of 2 pounds attached via pulley to the Gardner-Wells tongs. Repeat SSEPs and MEPs to confirm the absence of stretch injury to the neural elements should be performed. Traction should be immediately removed if any abnormalities are noted on ION.

A shoulder bump or inflatable bean bag should be placed between the shoulder blades of the patient to improve extension and lordotic alignment of the neck. All bony prominences are evaluated and protected. The patient's arms should rest at their side with a sheet wrapped around the arm proximal to the elbow joint and tucked securely under the bed. The head and neck should be supported to prevent perioperative motion. The placement of an adhesive tape to the bilateral shoulders and placed taut onto the end of the bed can provide additional neck exposure, with the awareness that increased traction of the shoulder can lead to damage at the brachial plexus, in particular the C5 nerve root. Elevation of the head of the bed to 30° can also be considered to increase neck exposure for the surgeon and partial venous draining of the neck for decreased perioperative bleeding. Optimal patient positioning will assist the surgeon in obtaining critical lateral radiographs during the procedure.

Surgical Approach

After the neck has been properly sterilely prepped and draped, palpation of the surface anatomy of the neck is utilized to determine the approximate cervical vertebral level as noted earlier. The location of the carotid pulse should also be noted prior to incision. A transverse incision is made starting just laterally to the midline and extending to the medial aspect of the SCM. The skin and subcutaneous tissue is carefully incised with the knife, taking time to achieve hemostasis via electrocautery. The superficial dissection lacks an internervous plane, but the thin fibers of the platysma muscle, innervated in the superior aspect of the neck by the facial nerve, can be horizontally split using scissors without issue, focusing again on careful dissection and hemostasis as the platysma muscle can be very vascular. A blunt versus a sharp dissection of the platysma can be continued parallel to the longitudinal fibers as needed for tissue mobilization. Structures at risk include the external jugular vein and the 11th cranial nerve with excessive platysma retraction.[14]

A plane deep to the platysma is created and the SCM invested in the deep cervical fascia should be visualized at the lateral aspect of the dissection with the lateral aspects of the sternohyoid and sternothyroid muscles. The deep cervical fascia over the SCM is incised using a knife or dissecting scissors with the surgeon's finger sweeping the SCM laterally and careful retraction of the sternohyoid and sternothyroid muscles, and underlying the trachea and esophagus medially. Blunt retractors should be placed under the minimum amount of tension both medially and laterally to prevent injury to important neck structures.

Next, the carotid sheath containing the carotid artery, internal jugular vein, and the vagus nerve is identified. The carotid pulse is once again palpated to confirm the correct location of dissection. The pretracheal fascia is encountered and incised medial to the carotid sheath and lateral to the thyroid cartilage, trachea, and esophagus. Care must be taken to look for the superior and inferior thyroid arteries which connect from the carotid sheath to the thyroid medially, particularly when the dissection is at or above the C3-4 level. Once the pretracheal fascia is incised, blunt dissection continues in the same plane deep to the carotid sheath. The surgeon must confirm the lateral location of the carotid sheath via carotid pulse palpation and palpation of the bony cervical vertebra at the medial aspect of the plane of dissection.

A careful retraction of both the carotid sheath laterally and the thyroid, esophagus, and trachea medially is performed as the longus colli muscle is identified. The cervical vertebra along with the vertebral discs can be identified as well. The normal anatomy of the cervical spine has the vertebral discs protruding anterior in relation to the bony vertebrae, but this relationship can be distorted with degenerative disc disease, trauma to the vertebrae and/or disc, or osseous abnormalities due to neoplastic or infectious processes. Referral to preoperative imaging may be needed to determine approximate level of the cervical spine with subsequent confirmation intraoperatively. The ALL can be seen in the midline. Of note, the cervical sympathetic chain lies just lateral to the cervical vertebra at this depth of dissection. A hemostat grabbing the longus colli muscle is placed and an intraoperative radiograph is taken to confirm the correct level of surgery. Alternatively, a spinal needle can be placed into the intervertebral disc for level confirmation (Fig. 2.1).

Once the correct cervical vertebral level has been identified via lateral radiograph and marked in the dissection, the longus colli muscle fascia can either be incised medially with sharp knife, scissor dissection, or using electrocautery. The authors prefer precise dissection with use of bipolar electrocautery to lift the longus colli off the vertebrae. Local retraction of the longus colli muscle over the operative cervical vertebrae does not lead to muscle denervation as the muscle is segmentally innervated.[5] For preparation of the corpectomy, further superior and inferior dissection, elevation, and retraction of the longus colli muscle is needed until the suitable surgical exposure is achieved. At this point, the authors prefer using the self-retaining retractors to provide continued exposure and the appropriate amount of retraction of the surrounding structures. After placement of blade-retractors, the endotracheal tube should briefly be deflated and re-inflated to decrease tension and pressure to the surrounding airway structures. Small 1–2 pound weights can be attached to the retracting apparatus to provide stability while performing the corpectomy, but other stabilizing devices can be used as well.

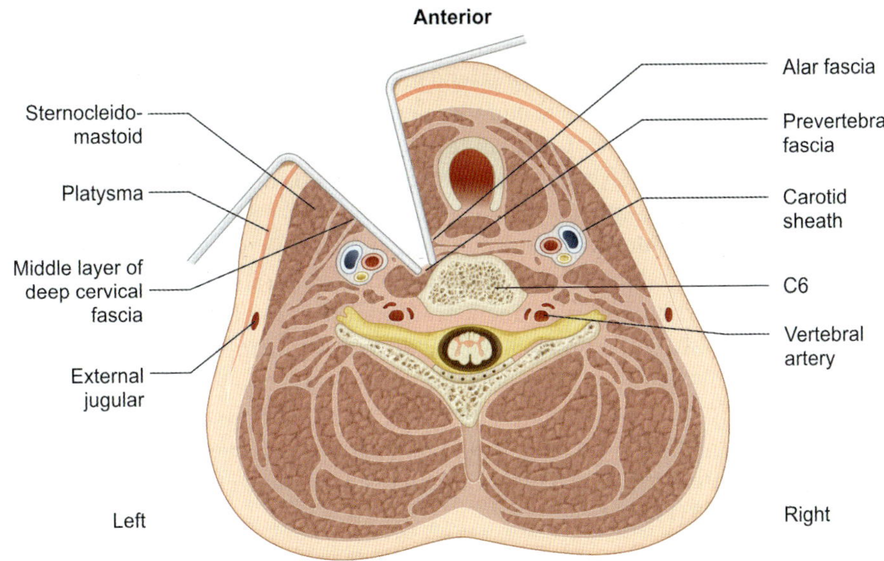

Fig. 2.1: The Smith-Robinson anterior cervical approach exploits the interval between the sternocleidomastoid and strap muscles. Dissection proceeds through deep cervical fascia medial to the carotid sheath.
Source: Rothman-Simeone, The Spine, 6th edition, Chapter 41.

Disc Excision

Removal of the vertebral discs surrounding the vertebral body being excised is performed. First, the discs are incised through the outer annulus fibrosus and into the softer nucleus pulposus. With significant degenerative disc disease, there may be a significant decrease in disc height possibly with surrounding endplate osteophytes that require removal with a rongeur. The remainder of the disc material is removed using either Kerrison or pituitary rongeurs and cervical curettes as needed. The superior and inferior endplate cartilage should be removed to promote bony fusion. The disc removal should proceed laterally until the uncovertebral joints are identified. Any further lateral dissection places the vertebral arteries at risk of injury. If there is any evidence of aberrant anatomy of the vertebral artery running medial to the pedicles, the corpectomy should be modified to avoid injury or aborted. Once all the disc material has been removed, the PLL should be evident at the floor of the dissection.

Vertebral Corpectomy

The corpectomy requires an understanding of the surrounding anatomy to prevent iatrogenic injury of the vertebral arteries laterally and underlying spinal canal. A midline trough is created using the Leksell rongeur and further expanded with use of a high-speed burr making sure to achieve the appropriate width of approximately 16 mm. This width allows for adequate decompression of the spinal cord with at least 5 mm margin of safety from the vertebral arteries (Fig. 2.2). At the level of the posterior cortex, once an adequate initial midline trough has been achieved and measured with a ruler, the operating microscope is used to improve the direct visualization of the corpectomy. The high-speed burr and irrigation help to break up the thicker bony endplates and posterior cortex.[15] Posteriorly, the decompression can be safely widened 2–3 mm as the decompression is now posterior to the location of the vertebral artery. Prior to this maneuver confirm the anterior posterior location of the vertebral artery in relationship to the posterior vertebral cortex.[16] Undercutting of the lateral margins to remove the posterior cortex of the vertebral body aids in the completion of the decompression (Fig. 2.3). It is important to carefully create a plane around the PLL and endplates using a small Kerrison rongeur and a nerve hook to aid in generating the potential space. Next, the foraminotomies are performed in a similar fashion removing the obstructing ligamentous tissue until the nerve probe can easily traverse toward the medial wall of the pedicle.

Throughout the corpectomy process, it is important to take time to confirm that the resection follows the midline raphe and is symmetrical. While this assessment is taking place, the SSEPs and MEPs can be taken to monitor neurologic function. In the instance of OPLL, gentle resection using a curette in a layer-by-layer fashion with careful, measured effort can allow for a successful and safe decompression.

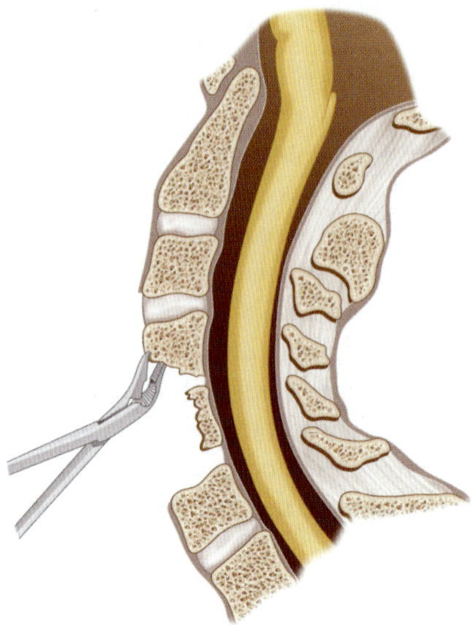

Fig. 2.2: Following discectomies cranial and caudal to the vertebral body, bony resection proceeds with the use of a Leksell rongeur followed by a high-speed burr. Care is taken to also create a docking site on the cranial vertebra for graft placement.
Source: Rothman-Simeone, The Spine, 6th edition, Chapter 41.

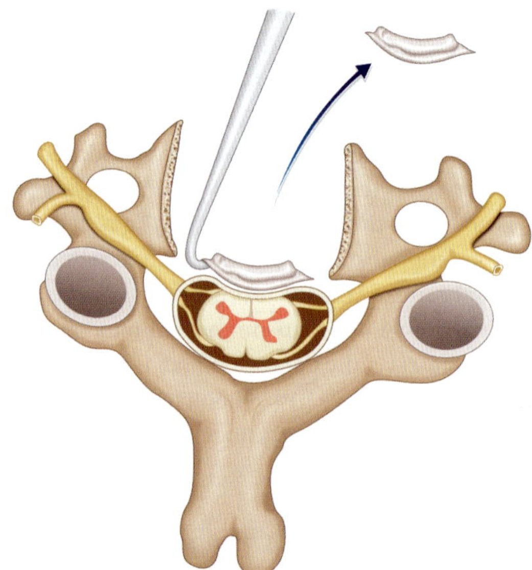

Fig. 2.3: Following resection of the vertebral body to the posterior cortex, this can then be thinned and removed with a combination of right angle curettes and Kerrison rongeurs to complete the decompression.
Source: Rothman-Simeone, The Spine, 6th edition, Chapter 41.

With OPLL, as much of the ligament should be removed as possible as remnants of it can lead to recurrence of symptoms postoperatively. Once the corpectomy is completed, hemostasis is achieved with the use of a thrombin-impregnated sealants and collagen matrices.

Strut Graft Preparation and Placement

The preparation of the recipient site for the graft starts with proper contouring of the bony endplates. Cancellous bone should be exposed to assist in the graft being incorporated into the site. The recipient site of the strut allograft or autograft needs to have posterior lip to prevent the graft from being tamped too far posteriorly and damaging the spinal cord. A depth gauge can be used to measure the appropriate depth of the graft, with a ruler measurement of the lateral width to compare to the graft.

Attention to the graft is then undertaken. If autograft is used, the graft will be harvested from the iliac crest to an approximate size of the vertebral trough. The graft must be meticulously shaped and sculpted to have an appropriate fit within the recipient site. The graft should have its depth undersized about 2–3 mm to prevent abutment of the spinal cord. Furthermore, a proper fit of the graft can provide indirect decompression of the nerve roots.

Distraction is applied to the vertebral trough to allow placement of the graft. This can be achieved using the Gardner-Wells tongs if already being utilized versus a Caspar pin distractor. Approximately 20 pounds of inline axial traction is placed on the cervical spine to provide the space for graft placement. Final length measurements of the recipient site are done and more Gelfoam is placed around the perimeter. Now, the graft should be assessed once more for proper dimensions in the axial, coronal, and sagittal plane. An undersized graft displaces anteriorly and results in residual kyphosis. An oversized graft can result in excessive traction and iatrogenic neurologic injury.

Placement of the graft necessitates complete control with proper instrumentation such as a Kelly clamp. After seating in the cranial docking site, the graft is tamped slowly into place while under distraction. Often, the correct fit requires multiple revisions of the graft, correcting height, length, and depth appropriately. The neck can be ranged in flexion and extension while under distraction to determine relative stability. The graft must be inserted with enough space for proper anterior plating and fixation. As soon as satisfactory fit of the strut graft is achieved, traction is slowly removed and another round of SSEPs and MEPs should be taken to ensure no nerve injury has occurred (Fig. 2.4).

Anterior Plating and Fixation

The surgeon then decides the appropriate instrumentation. Anterior plating reduces the risk of graft migration, nonunion, and duration of postoperative immobilization. The type of plate and screw fixation can allow for either a fixed, rigid construct or

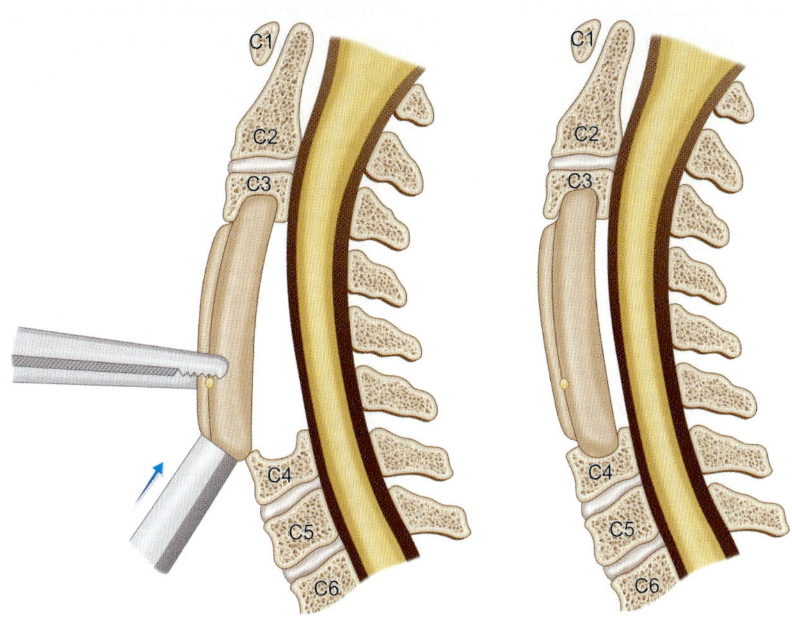

Fig. 2.4: Example of a C4 corpectomy requiring strut graft placement between C3 and C5. A docking site should be created in the cranial vertebra, following placement, the caudal aspect of the graft can then be carefully tamped into position.
Source: Rothman-Simeone, The Spine, 6th edition, Chapter 41.

a more load-sharing, and dynamic construct. This decision is made based on the patient's comorbidities and quality of bone stock. The goal is to obtain the best possible fusion of the graft. Screws, typically 4 mm in size, are placed in the vertebra above and below the corpectomy site. The smallest plate fixation possible offers the lowest risk of hardware failure and minimizes the risk of damaging the surrounding vertebral discs. Proper screw length and hardware placement should be confirmed via fluoroscopy or intraoperative lateral radiograph.

Wound Closure/Postoperative Care

The wound is closed in layers and a drain is placed in the wound prior to closure to prevent postoperative hematoma collection with most drains being removed on the following day. The patient receives a hard cervical collar to be worn for approximately 6 weeks postoperatively until follow-up with transition into a soft collar for another 2 weeks. Postoperative venous thromboembolism prophylaxis includes early ambulation and pneumatic compression devices. Anti-inflammatory medication is held for 6 weeks postoperatively and the patient is strongly advised to abstain from smoking due to risk of pseudarthrosis.

OUTCOMES

Fusion rates for ACCF approach, 95% for single or two level surgery with 87% of patients having resolution of symptoms such as imbalance, hand clumsiness, and arm weakness.[17,18] Successful outcomes following ACCF have been shown to depend on a number of preoperative variables. Duration of symptoms, age, preoperative functional status as noted by the modified Japanese Orthopaedic Association (mJOA) score and gait impairment, along with smoking status and psychological comorbidities have been shown to be predictive of outcomes.[19,20] Younger (<50 years old) nonsmoking patients with shorter (<3 months) durations of myelopathic symptoms have the highest probability of a successful outcome.[21] It is important to stress to patients, perioperatively, that smoking has consistently been a modifiable negative risk factor to fusion rates following ACCF and ACDF.[22]

COMPLICATIONS

Postoperative Epidural Hematoma/Airway Compromise

Ranging from 0.2% to 1.9% incidence in the literature, postoperative hematoma impinging on the spinal cord and airway is a rare, but potentially devastating complication following ACCF.[23] Risk factors for hematoma include increased age, history of a bleeding disorder, and impaired preoperative ambulation.[24] Careful observation of the wound postoperatively and close monitoring of wound drain output aid in prevention. If there is a high risk of postoperative hematoma formation, the surgeon may consider keeping a patient intubated until postoperative day 1.

DYSPHAGIA

Dysphagia is a common complaint following ACCF, especially with multilevel procedures and older patients.[25] Many patients will express a difficulty in eating solid foods postoperatively, so a soft diet should be started and advanced to solid foods as tolerated. Local analgesic throat sprays may be helpful in the immediate postoperative period. Specific types of instrumentation or grafting have not been shown to be correlated with postoperative dysphagia.

Recurrent Laryngeal Nerve Injury

Recurrent laryngeal nerve injury is a common complication with an incidence cited as high as 12% in some studies.[26] The RLN is usually damaged due to traction injury during the surgical approach, but more distal levels place the nerve at higher risk, particularly with right-sided dissection. While the left-sided approach is recommended by the authors, no statistically significant evidence in the literature proves that laterality places the RLN at increased risk for injury.[16] Patients will postoperatively complain of voice hoarseness or dysphonia.

Neurologic Injury

Patient positioning, corpectomy, and graft placement all can cause spinal cord injury without careful attention to technique. C5 is the most commonly injured nerve during ACCF.[27] Preoperative assessment of myelopathic symptoms and review of imaging to assess the overall cervical spine alignment and degree of spinal cord compression should help guide the degree of traction and neck extension that the patient can tolerate intraoperatively. Regular utilization of SSEPs and MEPs, especially during traction and graft placement, is the key to avoid neurologic injury during the procedure.

Graft Failure

With increased (three or greater) levels of decompression and corpectomy, the union rate of the graft material decreases below 50%. In cases where a three-level corpectomy or greater is indicated, the authors recommend supplemental posterior instrumentation and fusion. Similarly, a lack of proper fit can lead to graft migration with an incidence that increases with levels of surgery. Fusions that are noninstrumented have been shown to have increased rates of nonunion and graft migration as well. Meticulous graft contouring and recipient site preparation are critical to successful union.

Vertebral Artery Injury

Injury to the vertebral artery is another rare and severe complication that can occur during ACCF. Ranging from 0.5% to 1.0% incidence, vertebral artery injuries can occur due to retractor placement or direct injury from the high-speed burr. An anomalous route of the vertebral artery is a common association with injury. Direct tamponade often resolves the bleeding. Up to 5% of patients will suffer permanent neurologic deficits following injury.[28] Careful use of the high-speed burr and periodic assessment of the midline trough width, taking care to remain orthogonal during the corpectomy is critical to preventing this dangerous complication.

CASE PRESENTATION

A 67-year-old male presented with progressive hand weakness, upper extremity paresthesias, loss of dexterity, and gait dysfunction. He had been treated with comprehensive nonoperative management including physical therapy and anti-inflammatory medications. On physical examination, he is noted to have marked wrist extensor and hand intrinsic weakness. He is also found to have long tract signs including positive Hoffman's reflex bilaterally and hyperreflexia. The patient is noted to have a wide-based, unsteady gait consistent with myelopathy.

Radiographic imaging was notable for multilevel cervical spondylosis, disc degeneration, and kyphosis. MRI shows cord compression at C4-5 and C5-6 with retrovertebral compression behind the C5 body. T2-weighted imaging also demonstrates myelomalacia at these levels as well (Fig. 2.5). The patient consented to a C5 corpectomy with C4-6 anterior fusion. This was performed in standard fashion using iliac crest allograft. At 3-month follow-up, the patient noted improvements in balance and gait as well as mild improvements in hand strength and function (Fig. 2.6).

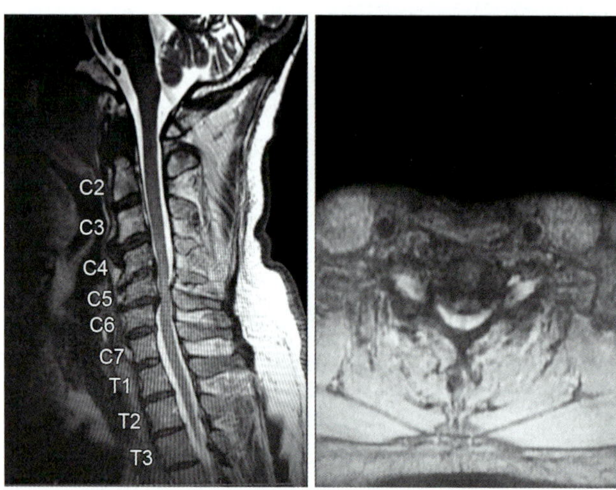

Fig. 2.5: Lateral T2-weighted MRI showing cord compression from C4-5 to C5-6 and myelomalacia with increased cord signal intensity at these levels. Axial T2 MRI at the level of the C5 body demonstrates retrovertebral cord compression.

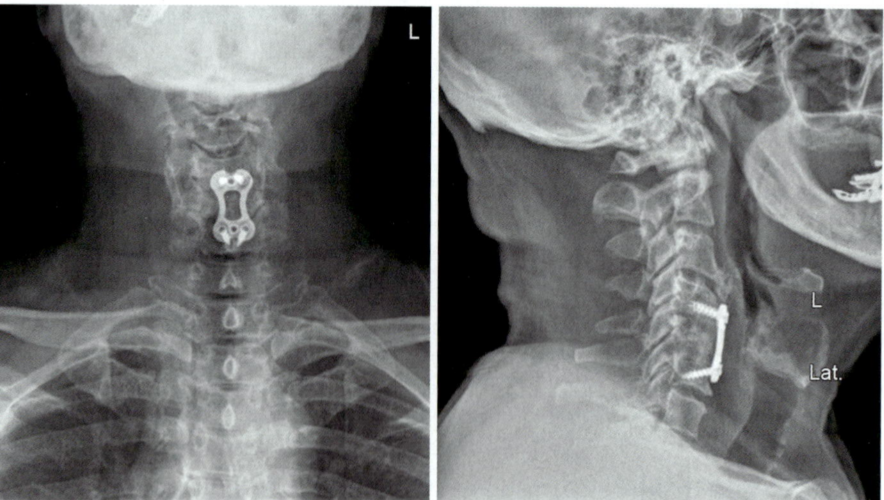

Fig. 2.6: A follow-up imaging at 3 months showed solid incorporation of the structural bone graft following C5 corpectomy and C4-6 anterior cervical fusion.

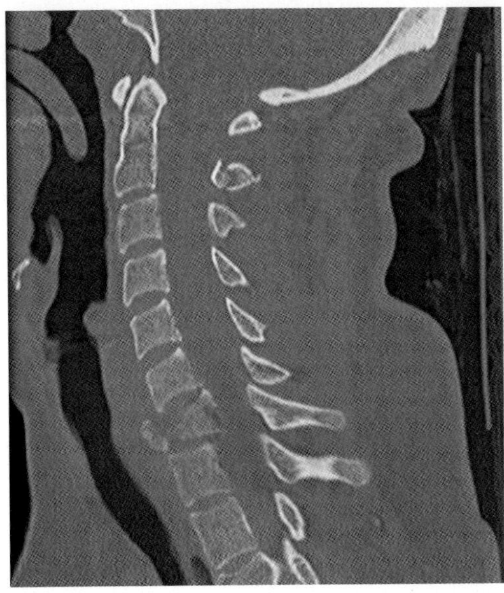

Fig. 2.7: Midsagittal computed tomography demonstrating a C7 burst fracture.

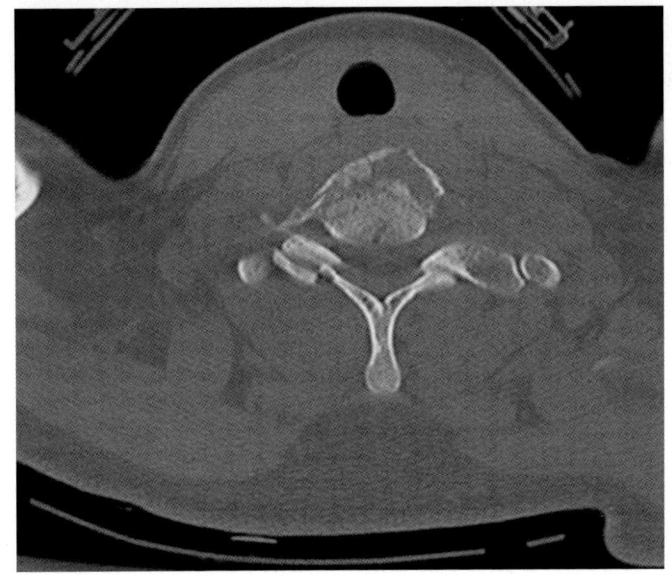

Fig. 2.8: Axial imaging at C7.

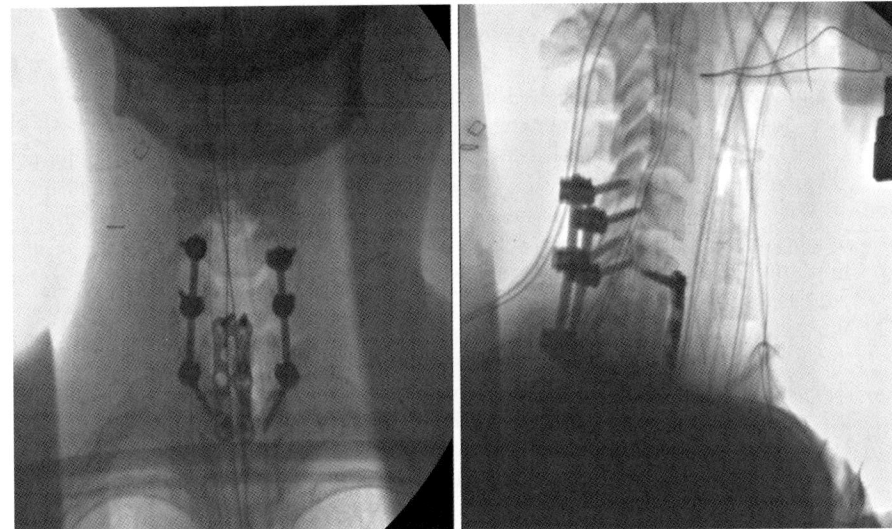

Fig. 2.9: Postoperative anteroposterior and lateral images showing a corpectomy at C7 with anterior plate fixation between C6 and T1 and posterior fixation spanning from C5 to T1.

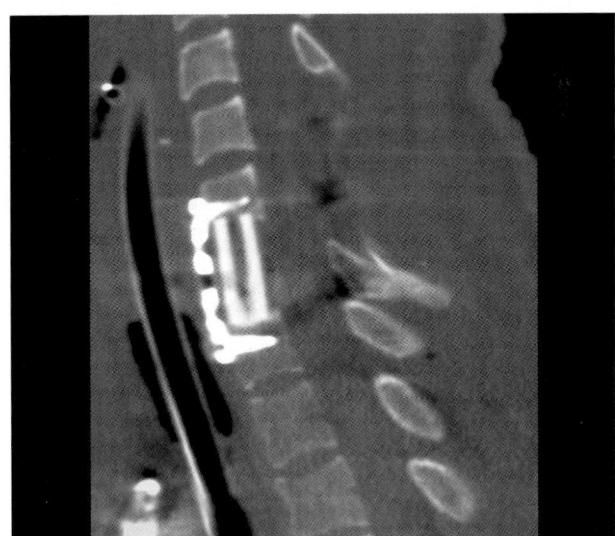

Fig. 2.10: Postoperative sagittal CT showing restoration of alignment and removal of posterior bony compression.
Courtesy: Dr. Alexander R Vaccaro.

Case Presentation

Anand Segar, Tyler Kreitz

This 37-year-old male presents after a shallow river diving accident. He sustained an axial load to his head. On examination, he was found to be an American Spinal Injury Association (ASIA) A with a motor level at T1. He had no other injuries.

Imaging revealed an AO A4 burst type fracture of C7. A CT scan showed an AO A4 burst fracture at C7 with lamina fractures at C5 and C6. An MRI (A CT scan) showed cord compression and edema behind the C7 vertebral body (Figs. 2.7 to 2.10).

REFERENCES

1. Johnson RM, Hart DL, Simmons EF, et al. Cervical orthoses. A study comparing their effectiveness in restricting cervical motion in normal subjects. J Bone Joint Surg Am. 1977;59(3):332-9.
2. Chiu WC, Haan JM, Cushing BM, et al. Ligamentous injuries of the cervical spine in unreliable blunt trauma patients: incidence, evaluation, and outcome. J Trauma. 2001;50(3):457-63. Discussion at 464.
3. Chen J, Wang W, Han G, et al. MR investigation in evaluation of chronic whiplash alar ligament injury in elderly patients. Zhong Nan Da Xue Xue Bao Yi Xue Ban. 2015;40(1): 67-71.
4. Pal GP, Routal RV, Saggu SK. The orientation of the articular facets of the zygapophyseal joints at the cervical and upper thoracic region. J Anat. 2001;198(Pt 4):431-41.
5. Hoppenfeld S, deBoer P, Buckley R. Surgical Exposures in Orthopaedics: The Anatomic Approach (Hoppenfeld, Surgical Exposures in Orthopaedics), 4th edition.
6. Pait TG, Killefer JA, Arnautovic KI. Surgical anatomy of the anterior cervical spine: the disc space, vertebral artery, and associated bony structures. Neurosurgery. 1996;39(4):769-76.
7. Walker HK. Cranial nerve XI: The spinal accessory nerve. In: Walker HK, Hall WD, Hurst JW (Eds). Clinical Methods: The History, Physical, and Laboratory Examinations, 3rd edition. Boston, MA: Butterworths; 1990.
8. Hartmann S, Tschugg A, Obernauer J, et al. Cervical corpectomies: Results of a survey and review of the literature on diagnosis, indications, and surgical technique. Acta Neurochir (Wien). 2016;158(10):1859-67.
9. Medow JE, Trost G, Sandin J. Surgical management of cervical myelopathy: Indications and techniques for surgical corpectomy. Spine J Off J North Am Spine Soc. 2006;6(6 Suppl):233S-41S.
10. Sugawara T. Anterior cervical spine surgery for degenerative disease: a review. Neurol Med Chir (Tokyo). 2015;55(7):540-6.
11. Ozgen S, Naderi S, Ozek MM, et al. A retrospective review of cervical corpectomy: Indications, complications and outcome. Acta Neurochir (Wien). 2004;146(10):1099-105. Discussion at 1105.
12. Ajiboye RM, Zoller SD, Sharma A, et al. Intraoperative neuromonitoring for anterior cervical spine surgery: What Is the evidence? Spine. 2017;42(6):385-93.
13. Shan J, Jiang H, Ren D, et al. Anatomic relationship between right recurrent laryngeal nerve and cervical fascia and its application significance in anterior cervical spine surgical approach. Spine. 2017;42(8):E443-7.
14. Azar FM, Canale ST, Beaty JH (Eds). Campbell's Operative Orthopaedics, 4-Volume Set, 13th edition.
15. Wang T, Tian X-M, Liu S-K, et al. Prevalence of complications after surgery in treatment for cervical compressive myelopathy: a meta-analysis for last decade. Medicine (Baltimore). 2017;96(12):e6421.
16. Miscusi M, Bellitti A, Peschillo S, et al. Does recurrent laryngeal nerve anatomy condition the choice of the side for approaching the anterior cervical spine? J Neurosurg Sci. 2007;51(2):61-4.
17. Emery SE, Bohlman HH, Bolesta MJ, et al. Anterior cervical decompression and arthrodesis for the treatment of cervical spondylotic myelopathy. Two to seventeen-year follow-up. J Bone Joint Surg Am. 1998;80(7):941-51.
18. Jamjoom A, Williams C, Cummins B. The treatment of spondylotic cervical myelopathy by multiple subtotal vertebrectomy and fusion. Br J Neurosurg. 1991;5(3):249-55.
19. Tetreault LA, Kopjar B, Vaccaro A, et al. A clinical prediction model to determine outcomes in patients with cervical spondylotic myelopathy undergoing surgical treatment: data from the prospective, multi-center AOSpine North America study. J Bone Joint Surg Am. 2013;95(18):1659-66.
20. Kanellopoulos GK, Kato H, Hsu CY, et al. Spinal cord ischemic injury. Development of a new model in the rat. Stroke. 1997;28(12):2532-8.
21. Pumberger M, Froemel D, Aichmair A, et al. Clinical predictors of surgical outcome in cervical spondylotic myelopathy. Bone Jt J. 2013;95-B(7):966-71.
22. Hilibrand AS, Fye MA, Emery SE, et al. Impact of smoking on the outcome of anterior cervical arthrodesis with interbody or strut-grafting. J Bone Joint Surg Am. 2001;83-A(5):668-73.
23. Palumbo MA, Aidlen JP, Daniels AH, et al. Airway compromise due to wound hematoma following anterior cervical spine surgery. Open Orthop J. 2012;6:108.
24. Lim S, Kesavabhotla K, Cybulski GR, et al. Predictors for airway complications following single- and multilevel anterior cervical discectomy and fusion. Spine. 2017;42(6):379-84.
25. Nagoshi N, Tetreault L, Nakashima H, et al. Risk factors for and clinical outcomes of dysphagia after anterior cervical surgery for degenerative cervical myelopathy: results from the AOSpine International and North America Studies. J Bone Joint Surg Am. 2017;99(13):1069-77.
26. Wu B, Song F, Zhu S. Reasons of dysphagia after operation of anterior cervical decompression and fusion. Clin Spine Surg. 2017;30(5):E554-9.
27. Ikenaga M, Shikata J, Tanaka C. Radiculopathy of C-5 after anterior decompression for cervical myelopathy. J Neurosurg Spine. 2005;3(3):210-7.
28. Lunardini DJ, Eskander MS, Even JL, et al. Vertebral artery injuries in cervical spine surgery. Spine J Off J North Am Spine Soc. 2014;14(8):1520-5.

CHAPTER

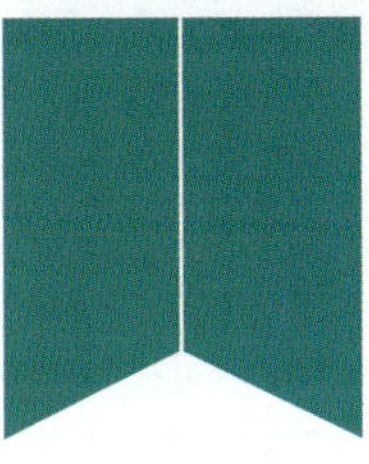

3

Cervical Total Disc Arthroplasty

Hannah Kirby, Patrick Morrissey, Nelson Saldua

ANATOMY

The cervical spine is comprised of seven vertebra with fibrocartilaginous intervertebral discs situated between each segment from C2 to C7. These discs are comprised of a tough outer covering of radially oriented collagen fibers known as the annulus fibrosus which surrounds the softer nucleus pulposus comprised mainly of water and a loose collagen fiber network. The annulus fibrosus is intertwined with both the anterior and posterior longitudinal ligament, which serve as the dorsal and ventral borders of the intervertebral space. The lateral borders of this space are defined by the uncinate processes, which extend from the lateral aspect of the superior endplates, creating a cup-like shape and articulating with the inferolateral border of the superior vertebral body. These articulations are called the uncovertebral joints. The sagittal depths of the cervical vertebral bodies average approximately 14 mm, but variability does exist and should be kept in mind during decompression.[1]

Lateral to the uncovertebral joints are the transverse foramen anteriorly and the lateral masses more posteriorly. The mean distance from the medial aspect of the uncovertebral joint to the medial aspect of the transverse foramen has been reported as 5.4 mm on the right side of all normal vertebrae and 5.7 mm on the left.[2] The vertebral artery typically travels within this foramen, with the average distance between the uncinate process and medial border of the vertebral artery being only 2 mm.[3] One must appreciate this important relationship during decompression, taking care not to venture lateral to the uncinate process which could result in an iatrogenic vertebral artery injury.

The neural foramen at each level is bordered superiorly and inferiorly by the pedicles of the adjacent vertebral bodies, anteromedially by the uncovertebral joints, and posterolaterally by the facet joints. There are eight cervical nerve roots, with each root exiting the spinal canal though the neural foramen above its corresponding numbered pedicle, with the exception of the C8 root, which exits above T1.

Other important neural structures are the sympathetic plexus and the recurrent laryngeal nerves. The sympathetic plexus lies on top of the longus colli muscle, which sits ventral to the vertebral column. The plexus can be damaged with poor retractor placement or excessive retraction. The recurrent laryngeal nerves run on either side of the trachea in the tracheoesophageal groove. There is more constant anatomy of the recurrent laryngeal nerve on the left side as it loops under the arch of the aorta, making this side the preferred approach for anterior cervical spine surgery[4] although nerve injury rates have been shown to be similar for both left and right side approaches.

SURGICAL INDICATIONS

In general, the indications for total cervical disc arthroplasty (CDA) are similar to anterior cervial decompression and fusion (ACDF). Any patient with anterior pathology and near normal segmental motion can be a candidate for CDA after they have failed an appropriate course of nonoperative treatment to include activity modification, physical therapy, nonsteroidal anti-inflammatory drugs, and possibly selective nerve root blocks.

Cervical disc arthroplasty candidates should have normal cervical spinal alignment and mobility along with either radiculopathy or myelopathy caused by a disc herniation or foraminal osteophytes.[5-7] The Food and Drug Administration (FDA) has approved CDA for both one- and two-level applications (implant specific) with several prospective studies demonstrating equivalent and in some cases superior results compared with traditional ACDF.

Contraindications to CDA include more than three vertebral levels requiring treatment, instability (translation > 3 mm and/or >11° rotational difference to that of either adjacent level), known allergy to implant materials, posttraumatic vertebral body deficiency or deformity, facet joint degeneration, significant deformity, bridging osteophytes, disc height loss more than 50%, and absence of motion (<2°). Other contraindications include osteoporosis/osteopenia, prior surgery at the level to be treated, active malignancy, systemic disease [acquired immunodeficiency syndrome (AIDS), human immunodeficiency virus (HIV), hepatitis B or C, and insulin-dependent diabetes], other metabolic bone disease, renal failure, Paget's disease, rheumatoid arthritis, morbid obesity, pregnancy, active or prior cervical infection, and chronic corticosteroid use.[6,7]

Many patients who are candidates for ACDF are candidates for CDA. A retrospective review of 167 consecutive patients who underwent elective cervical spine surgery found that 43% of patients would be candidates for CDA and that this amount increased to 47% if treatment of adjacent-level degeneration was included.

SURGICAL TECHNIQUE

Prior to proceeding to the operating room, every patient indicated for a CDA should also be consented for the possibility of changing the plan to an ACDF. This is important because there are several intraoperative challenges that can preclude safe and effective implantation, the most important of these being radiographic visualization. As we will show later, clear C-arm images of the complete intervertebral space are required for accurate device implantation. This can be difficult at the lower cervical levels, particularly C6-7. While these levels may be clearly imaged in upright office radiographs, they will often be difficult to see intraoperatively despite optimal patient positioning. If unable to obtain adequate imaging during the procedure, the surgeon should abort the CDA in favor of an ACDF, which does not require detailed fluoroscopic imaging.

Anesthetic considerations are identical to those in ACDF with mean arterial pressures maintained above 85 mm Hg for all patients with a diagnosis of myelopathy. As with all cervical spine surgery, routine neuromonitoring is strongly recommended with both motor and sensory evoked potentials obtained throughout the procedure.

Patient positioning in the operating room is paramount to the success of CDA. The patient should be positioned supine on a radiolucent table in order to allow for both anteroposterior (AP) and lateral fluoroscopic imaging. Arms should be appropriately padded with gel rolls or foam and tucked at the side using a draw sheet while ensuring thumbs are pointed up. The shoulders should be taped down and secured to the bed with 3-inch silk tape, making sure the force vector is aimed toward the patient's feet. This serves to both stabilize the patient and improve sagittal visualization, allowing the more caudal levels to be clearly seen on fluoroscopy. The neck should be positioned in neutral rotation and with neutral lordosis. The authors suggest using an inflatable intravenous (IV) pressure bag placed in the interscapular region to allow for fine adjustments of sagittal alignment during the procedure should they be necessary. You may also choose to secure the head to the table by taping the chin or forehead to prevent intraoperative rotation.

The skin incision should be made according to standard palpable landmarks. The hyoid bone is typically at C3, thyroid cartilage is at C4-5, and the cricoid cartilage is at C6. The skin incision should extend from just across midline to the medial border of the sternocleidomastoid. The approach is carried out in a manner similar to ACDF. The platysma is incised in line with the skin incision and a subplatysmal flap is developed bluntly. The interval between the sternocleidomastoid laterally and the strap muscles medially is identified and bluntly dissected with scissors. Occasionally, when operating on caudal cervical levels, the omohyoid muscle can preclude adequate exposure. Should this be the case, the muscle can be divided at its medial aspect with electrocautery, with no repair required at the conclusion of the procedure. The carotid sheath is identified by palpating the pulse and the entire sheath and its contents should be maintained laterally. The pretracheal fascia is divided within this interval, exposing the prevertebral fascia overlying the longus colli musculature and the cervical spine. The prevertebral space is bluntly cleared with gentle finger sweeps both cranially and caudally and the prevertebral fascia is divided longitudinally. The vertebral bodies and intervertebral discs are easily identifiable with the overlying longus colli and anterior longitudinal ligament (ALL). The appropriate cervical level is identified with a lateral radiograph.

Once the appropriate level has been identified, the longus colli musculature is elevated to expose the disc space from uncus to uncus. A cranial and caudal dissection should expose at least the midpoint of the vertebral bodies above and below the operative level. Self-retaining radiolucent retractors are then placed under the elevated longus colli, being careful to avoid damaging the cervical sympathetic chain that overlies these muscles. It is important to minimize soft tissue trauma during this step to decrease the possibility of postoperative heterotopic ossification.

Once the operative level is exposed, Caspar pins are placed in the cranial and caudal vertebral bodies. The pin placement is extremely important and should be performed under fluoroscopic guidance. In the coronal plane, the pins should be placed perfectly midline. In the sagittal plane, they should be placed parallel to the endplates and at least 5 mm from the disc space to facilitate decompression and instrumentation (Fig. 3.1). A Caspar pin distractor is then placed to facilitate decompression and device implantation.

The decompression is performed with several important considerations. A thorough discectomy is required, removing all disc material and endplate cartilage; however, unlike the decompression in ACDF, particular attention is paid to preservation of the bony endplate structure. Maintaining the natural dome of the inferior endplate of the cranial vertebra and the symmetric upslope of the uncus on the superior endplate of the caudal vertebra will assist with device fit and segmental stability. If possible, small anterior osteophytes and bony overhang should be preserved. Following discectomy, the posterior longitudinal ligament is symmetrically released and decompression of the canal and foramen is carried out with the use of a Kerrison rongeur. The posterior uncinate process may be taken as part of the decompression, but the remainder should be left intact anteriorly.

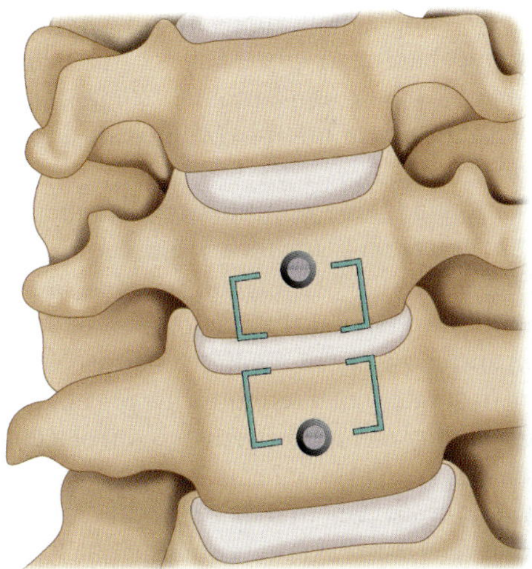

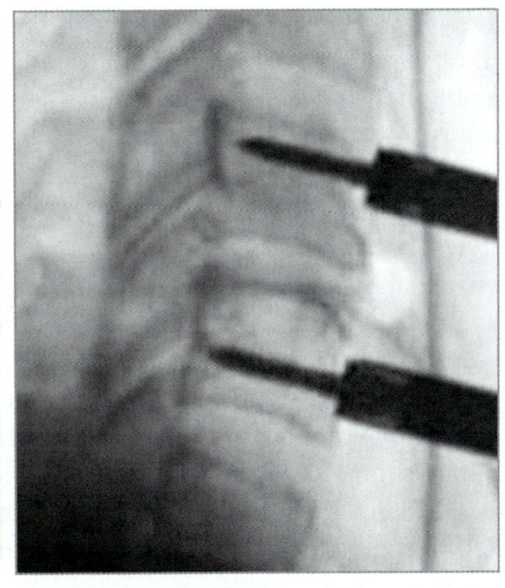

Fig. 3.1: Caspar pins should be placed in the center of the vertebral body on AP imaging (left) and parallel to the operative endplates (right), ensuring at least 5 mm of working distance from either endplate (AP: anteroposterior).

Once the decompression is complete, width and depth measurements are taken as per the manufacturer's recommended technique. The appropriately sized trial components are then placed under fluoroscopic guidance. Start the insertion with lateral fluoroscopy, ensuring that implant trajectory is in line with the disc space. Gently tap the trial into place, stopping once it is centered in the disc space. Release the Caspar pin distraction and assess trial size by comparing the operative disc height to the levels above and below, being careful not to overstuff the disc space. At this point, one should also confirm that the trial is appropriately centered on AP fluoroscopy.

Once satisfied with trial placement, reapply Caspar pin distraction and remove the trial. Assemble the device on the insertion handle as per the manufacturer's instruction and prepare for final implant placement. Again, insertion is performed under fluoroscopic guidance ensuring that the implant is in line with the disc space on the lateral radiograph. In addition to this radiographic check, also ensure that the insertion handle is perpendicular to the operating room table when viewed from the patient's feet to account for appropriate medial/lateral trajectory. Gently insert the implant according to the specific manufacturer's instructions. An ideally placed implant will fill the anterior-posterior diameter on the lateral radiograph and will be centered on the AP image (Fig. 3.2). If the implant is slightly smaller than the disc space on the lateral, ensure it is centered from front to back as opposed to being flush with the posterior aspect of the vertebral body. Once satisfied with implant position, remove distraction and take final fluoroscopic images.

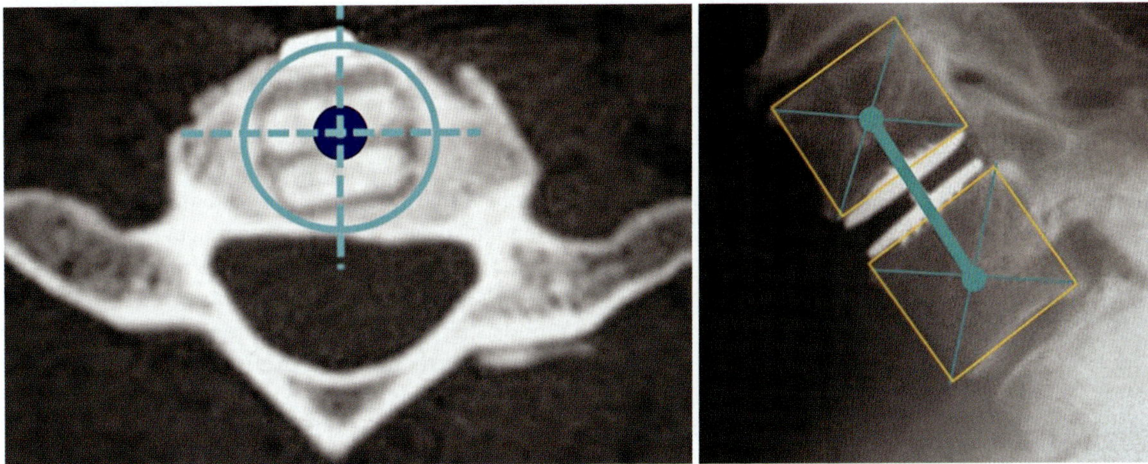

Fig. 3.2: Ideal implant positioning should be centered within the vertebral body. This is confirmed on AP and lateral fluoroscopy prior to conclusion of the case (AP: anteroposterior).

Careful attention is paid to ensure complete hemostasis, including the use of bone wax in Caspar pin tracts. A retropharyngeal drain often recommended overnight to lessen the likelihood of a postoperative hematoma. The platysmal and dermal layers are both closed with an absorbable braided suture and a monofilament suture is used for the skin. A postoperative cervical collar is not required, although a soft collar may be used initially for patient comfort for 1–2 weeks.

OUTCOMES

The widespread use of cervical total disc arthroplasty started with the BRYAN® Cervical Disc (Medtronic) in 2000. Many designs have followed, but the longest outcome data is on the Bryan prosthesis. The theoretical advantage of CDA is to maintain motion, with the hopes to avoid symptomatic adjacent segment disease which has been described as occurring at a rate of 2.9% per year.[8]

Sasso et al.[9] described 7–10 year follow-up for CDA, with the BRYAN® Cervical Disc (Medtronic), versus ACDF in a single-center randomized prospective trial. At 7 and 10 years of follow-up, both groups improved and maintained the improvement in comparison to their preoperative neck disability index (NDI) and Visual Analog Scale (VAS) neck/arm baseline scores. The NDI was significantly better for the CDA group versus the ACDF group at both time points; 8.6 and 21 at the 7-year follow-up and 8 and 15 at the 10-year follow-up, respectively ($p = 0.0138$ and $p = 0.0485$). At the 7-year follow-up, the VAS neck and arm scores were also significantly different favoring CDA but became statistically insignificant at 10 years. At 10 years, the CDA group demonstrated a trend toward less reoperation due to adjacent segment disease as compared to the ACDF group. Two patients (9%) of the CDA group required operative interventions (one patient at an adjacent level and a second patient at a nonadjacent level), and eight patients (32%) of the ACDF group required reoperation (six at adjacent levels and two patients at nonadjacent levels). Overall surgical survivorship of the CDA group was 90.90 versus 68.0% in the ACDF group, but this difference was not significant.[9]

A recent meta-analysis of randomized controlled trials with a minimum of 2-year follow-up showed a significant different in reoperation rate of 6% (108 of 1,762) in the CDA group and 12% (171 of 1,472) in the ACDF group.[10] While this meta-analysis showed a significantly higher revision rate in the ACDF cohort, the authors caution interpretation of these results given the limited follow-up and heterogeneity of studies included. At this time, while CDA has been established as a safe alternative to ACDF in select patient populations, additional studies are needed to determine efficacy of one technique over the other.

COMPLICATIONS

Complications of anterior cervical spinal surgery can be divided into intraoperative, early, and late. The intraoperative risks of CDA are similar to ACDF with intraoperative complications including injuries to the esophagus, vertebral artery, and recurrent laryngeal nerve. Dural tears and spinal cord or nerve root injuries are also possible.[11] These adverse events can occur for various reasons including inappropriate retractor placement, inadvertent intraoperative trauma, poor preoperative planning, excessive lateral discectomy, and patient positioning.

All of these complications are rare, but can have devastating consequences. Esophageal injury has been reported in 0.2–0.4%[12-14] and can have mortality rates approaching 20% even when identified early. The incidence of vertebral artery injury was found to be 0.3% in a review of 1,976 patients undergoing anterior cervical surgery,[15] also with a high rate of additional systemic complications. The incidence of dural tear during anterior cervical spine surgery has been reported at 1–3.7%[16] with a study analyzing 1,223 anterior spinal surgery cases showing a rate of 1%.[17] Spinal cord injury has an incidence of 0.2–0.9%[13,16,18] with the risk minimized by the widespread implementation of intraoperative neuromonitoring.

Early and late postoperative complications include reintubation, dysphagia, dysphonia from recurrent laryngeal nerve injury, Horner's syndrome, and retropharyngeal hematoma requiring evacuation (1%).[19,20] Airway compromise, which can occur secondary to soft tissue edema, retropharyngeal hematoma, or airway reactivity is a life-threatening complication and should be immediately addressed by reintubation and then appropriate medical or surgical interventions. The prevalence of reintubation from all causes was 0.1% in a multicenter retrospective cohort of 8,887 patients undergoing anterior cervical spine surgery.[21]

The incidence of dysphagia varies widely from 28% to 57%[22-24] and is mostly self-limited with prolonged moderate to severe dysphagia reported in 1.3–4% of patients.[20,22] The incidence of dysphonia also varies in the literature, but most cases of recurrent laryngeal nerve injury recover with time. A persistent symptomatic vocal fold paresis ranges from 0.33 to 2.5%.[25,26]

For all of the complications above, both CDA and ACDF have similar risk profiles with no significant differences between the procedures.[19,20] However, there are unique complications for cervical total disc arthroplasty including implant malposition, heterotopic ossification, osteolysis, intraoperative prosthesis migration (1%), and overmilling of the vertebral body (1%) leading to implant subsidence.[20]

One group investigating the complications associated with the BRYAN® Cervical Disc (Medtronic) analyzed 96 disc arthroplasties in 74 patients. The perioperative complication rate was 6.2% per treated level. In one patient (1%) a retropharyngeal hematoma developed, requiring evacuation. Neurological worsening occurred in three patients. Intraoperative migration of the prosthesis was observed in one two-level case (1%), whereas delayed migration occurred in one patient with postoperative segmental kyphosis (1%). In another patient with severe postoperative segmental kyphosis, revision was required with a customized lordotic prosthesis. Heterotopic ossification and spontaneous fusion occurred in two cases (2%).[20] Several case reports of vertebral body osteolysis and fractured or dislocated implants have also been described, and while the consequences of such failure are potentially catastrophic, these events are fortunately very rare.[27,28]

CASE PRESENTATION

A 31-year-old female was involved in a motor vehicle accident with subsequent right arm pain that did not respond to 6 weeks of conservative treatment including physical therapy, anti-inflammatory medications, and injections. The examination demonstrated normal neck range of motion (ROM) with significant pain, a positive Spurling's sign, and 4/5 strength in the biceps on the right with a slightly decreased deep tendon reflex. She had no long tract findings and no subjective myelopathic complaints. A magnetic resonance imaging (MRI) demonstrated a right-sided disc herniation with compression of the spinal cord and exiting nerve root at C5-6 (Fig. 3.3). Cervical spine radiographs demonstrated preservation of cervical disc height, normal lordosis, and full ROM (Fig. 3.4).

The patient underwent an uncomplicated CDA at C5-6 (Figs. 3.5A to D). Six weeks postoperatively, the patient had complete resolution of arm pain, full strength, and normal neck ROM. 1-year follow-up radiographs demonstrated appropriate implant placement with no evidence of complications and no findings of adjacent segment degeneration (Fig. 3.6).

Case Presentation

Anand Segar, Tyler Kreitz

Cervical Disc Replacement

A 33-year-old female presents with bilateral C6 radiculopathy and weakness in wrist extension and minimal neck pain. She had failed nonoperative management and was adverse to a fusion procedure. Her X-rays showed a well-aligned spine with preserved disc space and minimal facet arthrosis. She was indicated for a C5/6 CDA (Figs. 3.7 to 3.11).

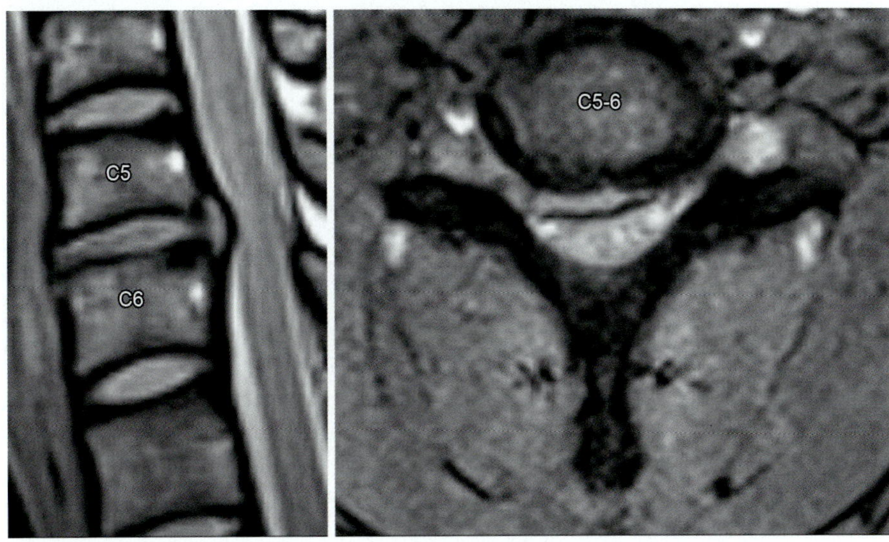

Fig. 3.3: Sagittal (left) and axial (right) MRI demonstrating an acute right-sided disc herniation at C5-6 with compression of both the spinal cord and the exiting nerve root. Overall disc height is maintained relative to the unaffected levels (MRI: magnetic resonance imaging).

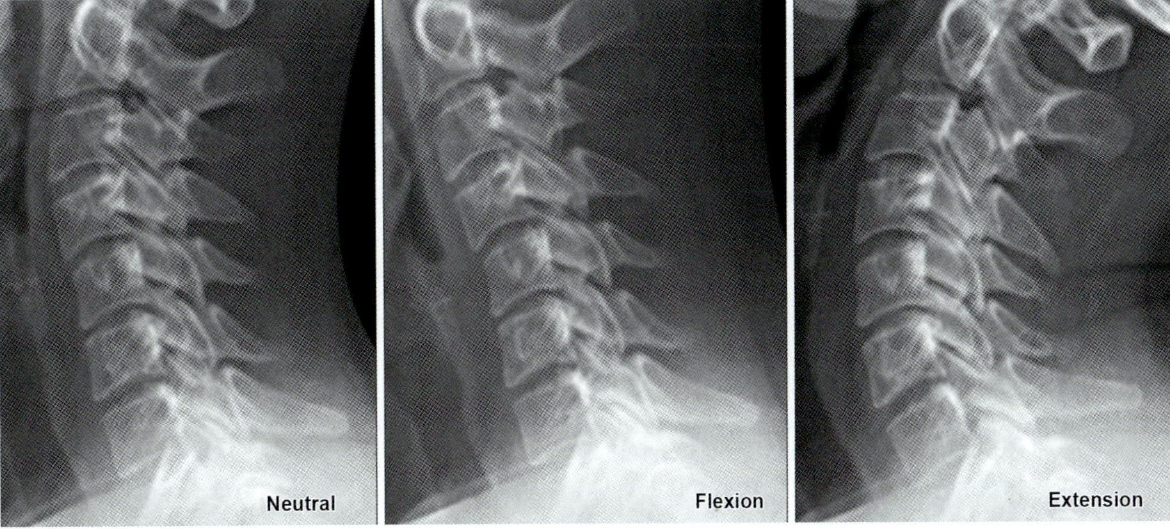

Fig. 3.4: Preoperative lateral cervical spine radiographs demonstrating minimal spondylosis, preservation of lordosis, and normal cervical spinal range of motion.

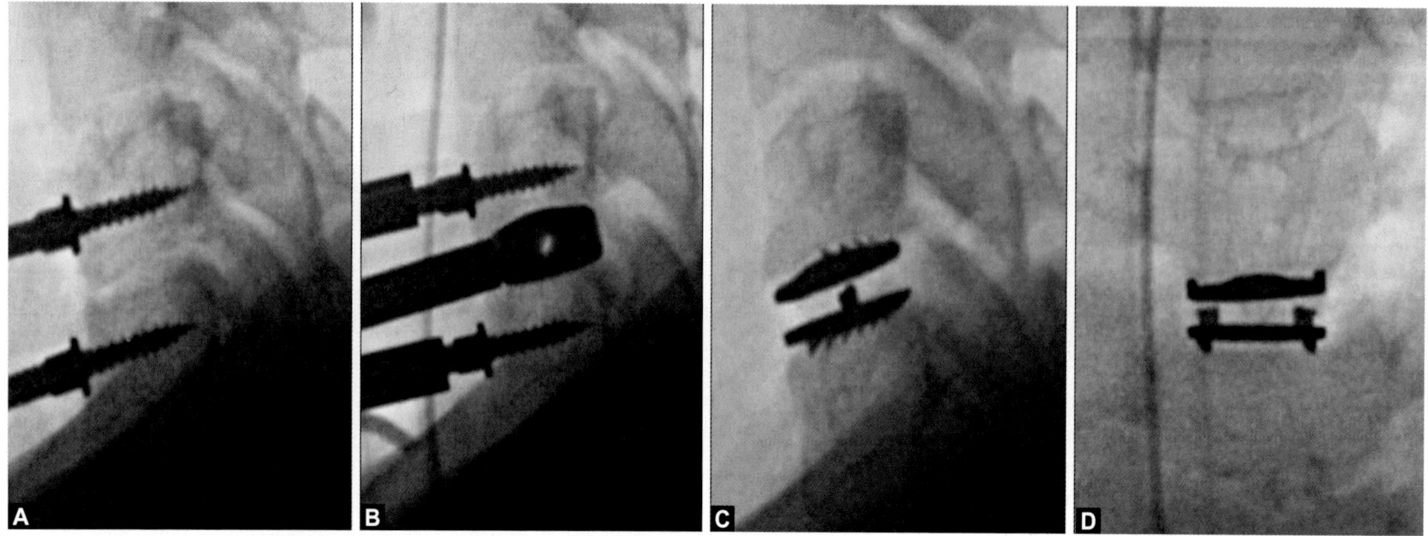

Figs. 3.5A to D: Intraoperative fluoroscopy demonstrating appropriate parallel Caspar pin placement (A) and trial insertion (B). Final lateral (C) and AP (D) radiographs demonstrate a well-centered implant with an implant height that is similar to the surrounding unaffected disc spaces (AP: anteroposterior).

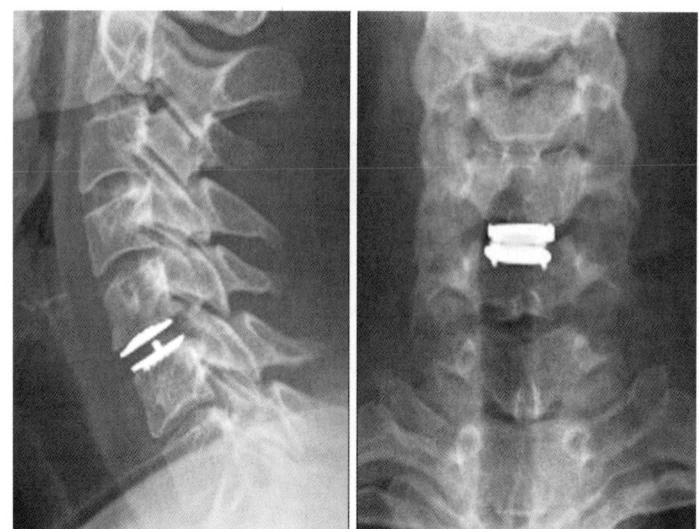

Fig. 3.6: Lateral (left) and AP (right) radiographs obtained at 1-year follow-up. Implant position is appropriately maintained and there is no evidence of adjacent segment degeneration (AP: anteroposterior).

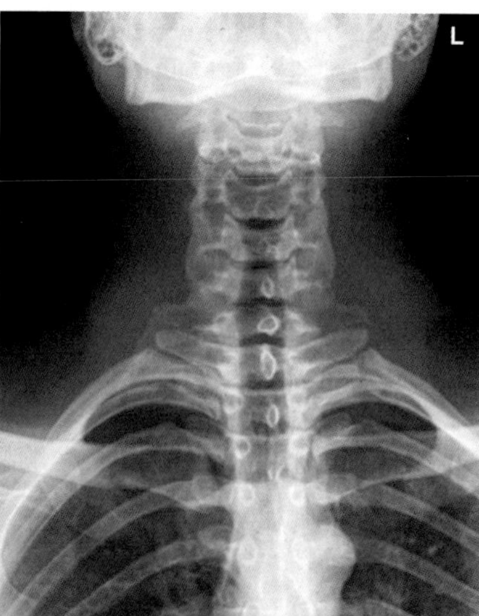

Fig. 3.7: Preoperative AP X-ray showing minimal uncovertebral arthrosis (AP: anteroposterior).

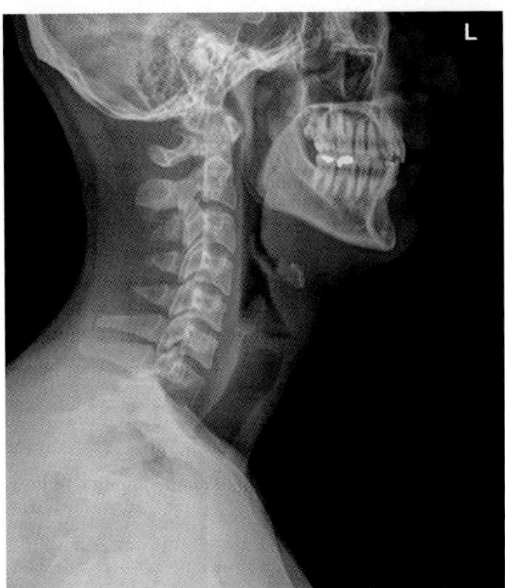

Fig. 3.8: Preoperative lateral X-ray showing minimal facet arthrosis, no listhesis, and preserved disc height.

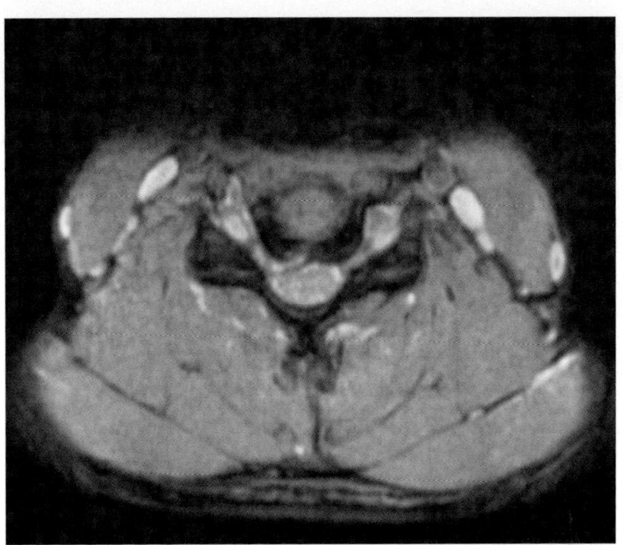

Fig. 3.9: Preoperative axial MR at C5/6 level image showing bilateral foramina stenosis with a right-sided herniated disc (MR: magnetic resonance).

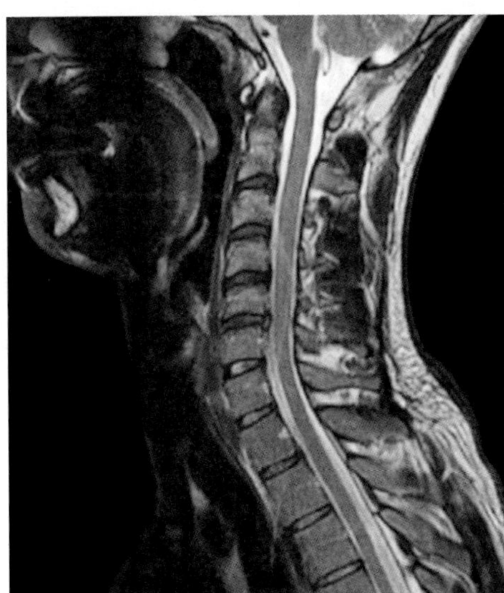

Fig. 3.10: Preoperative sagittal image showing no central stenosis or cord signal change.

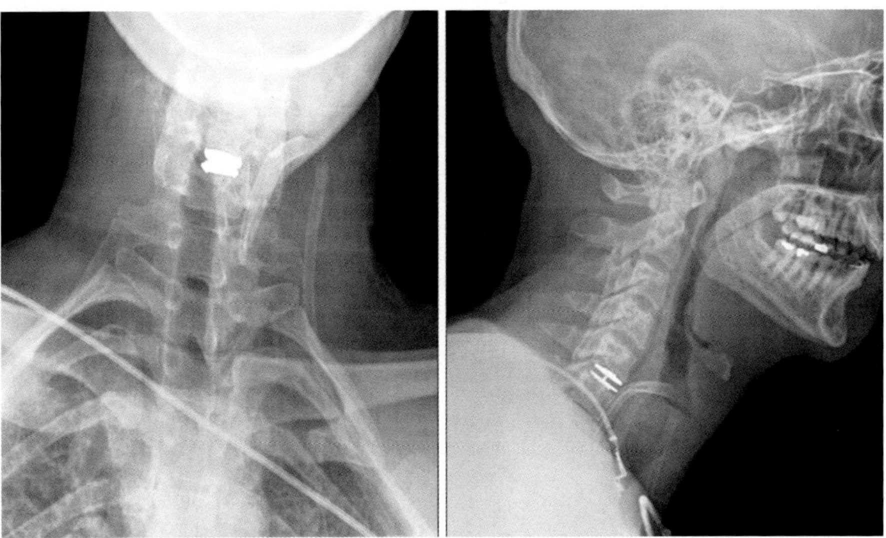

Fig. 3.11: Postoperative AP and lateral image demonstrating an implanted cervical arthroplasty at C5-6 in appropriate alignment.
Courtesy: Dr Alexander R Vaccaro.

REFERENCES

1. Ebraheim NA, Fow J, Xu R, et al. The vertebral body depths of the cervical spine and its relation to anterior plate-screw fixation. Spine (Phila Pa 1976). 1998;23(21):2299-302.
2. Curylo LJ, Mason HC, Bohlman HH, et al. Tortuous course of the vertebral artery and anterior cervical decompression: a cadaveric and clinical case study. Spine (Phila Pa 1976). 2000;25(22):2860-4.
3. Ebraheim NA, Reader D, Xu R, et al. Location of the vertebral artery foramen on the anterior aspect of the lower cervical spine by computed tomography. J Spinal Disord. 1997;10(4):304-7.
4. Ebraheim NA, Lu J, Skie M, et al. Vulnerability of the recurrent laryngeal nerve in the anterior approach to the lower cervical spine. Spine (Phila Pa 1976). 1997;22(22):2664-7.
5. Pracyk JB, Traynelis VC. Treatment of the painful motion segment. Spine (Phila Pa 1976). 2005;30(Suppl):S23-32.
6. Auerbach JD, Jones KJ, Fras CI, et al. The prevalence of indications and contraindications to cervical total disc replacement. Spine J. 2008;8(5):711-6.
7. McAfee PC. The indications for lumbar and cervical disc replacement. Spine J. 2004;4(6):S177-81.
8. Hilibrand AS, Carlson GD, Palumbo MA, et al. Radiculopathy and myelopathy at segments adjacent to the site of a previous anterior cervical arthrodesis. J Bone Joint Surg Am. 1999;81(4):519-28.
9. Sasso WR, Smucker JD, Sasso MP, et al. Long-term clinical outcomes of cervical disc arthroplasty. Spine (Phila Pa 1976). 2017;42(4):209-16.
10. Zhong Z-M, Zhu S-Y, Zhuang J-S, et al. Reoperation after cervical disc arthroplasty versus anterior cervical discectomy and fusion: a meta-analysis. Clin Orthop Relat Res. 2016;474(5):1307-16.
11. Daniels AH, Riew KD, Yoo JU, et al. Adverse events associated with anterior cervical spine surgery. J Am Acad Orthop Surg. 2008;16(12):729-38.
12. Orlando ER, Caroli E, Ferrante L. Management of the cervical esophagus and hypofarinx perforations complicating anterior cervical spine surgery. Spine (Phila Pa 1976). 2003;28(15):E290-5.
13. Tew JM, Mayfield FH. Complications of surgery of the anterior cervical spine. Clin Neurosurg. 1976;23:424-34.
14. Bertalanffy H, Eggert HR. Complications of anterior cervical discectomy without fusion in 450 consecutive patients. Acta Neurochir (Wien). 1989;99(1-2):41-50.
15. Burke JP, Gerszten PC, Welch WC. Iatrogenic vertebral artery injury during anterior cervical spine surgery. Spine J. 2005;5(5):508-14.
16. Emery SE, Bohlman HH, Bolesta MJ, et al. Anterior cervical decompression and arthrodesis for the treatment of cervical spondylotic myelopathy. Two to seventeen-year follow-up. J Bone Joint Surg Am. 1998;80(7):941-51.
17. Syre P, Bohman L-E, Baltuch G, et al. Cerebrospinal fluid leaks and their management after anterior cervical discectomy and fusion: a report of 13 cases and a review of the literature. Spine (Phila Pa 1976). 2014;39(16):E936-43.
18. Hilibrand AS, Schwartz DM, Sethuraman V, et al. Comparison of transcranial electric motor and somatosensory evoked potential monitoring during cervical spine surgery. J Bone Joint Surg Am. 2004;86-A(6):1248-53.
19. Goffin J, Van Calenbergh F, van Loon J, et al. Intermediate follow-up after treatment of degenerative disc disease with the Bryan Cervical Disc Prosthesis: Single-level and bi-level. Spine (Phila Pa 1976). 2003;28(24):2673-8.
20. Pickett GE, Sekhon LHS, Sears WR, et al. Complications with cervical arthroplasty. J Neurosurg Spine. 2006;4(2):98-105.
21. Nagoshi N, Fehlings MG, Nakashima H, et al. Prevalence and outcomes in patients undergoing reintubation after anterior cervical spine surgery: Results from the AOSpine North America Multicenter Study on 8887 patients. Glob Spine J. 2017;7(1_suppl):96S-102S.
22. Lee MJ, Bazaz R, Furey CG, et al. Risk factors for dysphagia after anterior cervical spine surgery: a two-year prospective cohort study. Spine J. 2007;7(2):141-7.
23. Smith-Hammond CA, New KC, Pietrobon R, et al. Prospective analysis of incidence and risk factors of dysphagia in spine surgery patients. Spine (Phila Pa 1976). 2004;29(13):1441-6.
24. Edwards CC, Karpitskaya Y, Cha C, et al. Accurate identification of adverse outcomes after cervical spine surgery. J Bone Joint Surg Am. 2004;86-A(2):251-6.
25. Jung A, Schramm J, Lehnerdt K, et al. Recurrent laryngeal nerve palsy during anterior cervical spine surgery: A prospective study. J Neurosurg Spine. 2005;2(2):123-7.
26. Apfelbaum RI, Kriskovich MD, Haller JR. On the incidence, cause, and prevention of recurrent laryngeal nerve palsies during anterior cervical spine surgery. Spine (Phila Pa 1976). 2000;25(22):2906-12.
27. Tumialán LM, Gluf WM. Progressive vertebral body osteolysis after cervical disc arthroplasty. Spine (Phila Pa 1976). 2011;36(14):E973-8.
28. Fan H, Wu S, Wu Z, et al. Implant failure of bryan cervical disc due to broken polyurethane sheath. Spine (Phila Pa 1976). 2012;37(13):E814-6.

CHAPTER

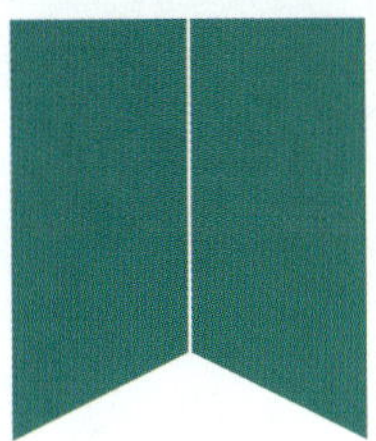

4

Cervical Laminoplasty

Andrew Wright, Patrick Morrissey, Alan Hilibrand

ANATOMY

There are many variations of the laminoplasty technique, but the goal is always the same—a posteriorly based decompression of the spinal cord with maintenance of the architecture of the posterior elements. Its advantages over laminectomy alone are additional stability and less postoperative kyphosis whereas its advantage over laminectomy and fusion is motion preservation. Typically, laminoplasty procedures require no postoperative immobilization as all three columns of the spine remain intact and there is no intrasegmental fusion taking place.

The lower cervical spine (C3–C7) has bony and ligamentous stabilizers. The distinct upsloping end-plates of the cervical spine and saucer-in-cup morphology of the uncovertebral joint are thought to resist posterior translation of the cephalad vertebra.[1] The addition of intervertebral disc, anterior longitudinal ligament, and posterior longitudinal ligament make up a very strong anterior discoligamentous complex. The posterior elements include the transverse processes, cervical pedicles, facet joints with their intervening lateral masses, lamina, spinous processes, interspinous ligaments, and supraspinous ligaments. The transverse processes and cervical pedicles intersect at the transverse foramen, which contains the vertebral artery. This provides protection to the important vertebral artery, but little in the way of subaxial spinal stability. As the cervical pedicle transitions to the lateral mass of its respective level, the lateral masses form the facet joint which are made up of superior and inferior articular processes of adjacent vertebrae. This zygapophyseal articulation functions as a bony constraint in the posterior cervical spine.

The cervical laminae arise from the posteromedial aspect of the lateral masses to converge and close the bony ring protecting the spinal cord. As the laminae converge at the midline, they form the spinous process. This spinous process acts as a bony attachment for the stout interspinous and supraspinous ligaments. The ligamentum flavum spans each interlaminar space in a noncontiguous manner providing thick soft-tissue coverage over the dorsal aspect of the dura in addition to serving as a soft tissue stabilizer in the posterior spine.

INDICATIONS

Cervical laminoplasty is indicated for the treatment of myelopathy caused by multilevel cervical stenosis. It has been described as a treatment for numerous etiologies including spondylosis, herniated nucleus pulposus, congenital spinal stenosis, ossification of the posterior longitudinal ligament, and several neuromuscular conditions. Patients who desire to avoid fusion and are not significantly affected by the neck pain may benefit from laminoplasty. An ideal patient presents with neutral or lordotic sagittal cervical alignment without instability on flexion-extension views, little to no neck pain, and multilevel disease.[2]

Laminoplasty allows retention of a bony bridge over the spinal cord and preservation of the posterior tension band with the resultant decrease in the incidence of post laminectomy kyphosis.[3] This allows for decreased scar tissue formation and better preservation of normal surgical landmarks which is beneficial should revision surgery become necessary.

TECHNIQUE

Patient positioning for cervical laminoplasty can be done on either a regular operating table with parallel chest rolls and pinions or on a Jackson spine frame with a padded headholder. Regardless of the bed of choice, it is important to ensure that the patient's neck can be adequately flexed to decrease shingling of the cervical lamina and allow for adequate laminar mobilization during the procedure. We routinely use intraoperative neurophysiologic monitoring to lessen the likelihood of neurologic injury during the procedure and recommend maintaining the mean arterial pressure above 85 mm Hg to ensure adequate spinal cord perfusion.

A standard midline posterior approach is performed while limiting lateral soft tissue dissection to prevent iatrogenic injury to the facet capsules. Once the target levels are exposed, the interspinous ligaments are removed to isolate each lamina. A side-cutting burr is then used to create a unilateral full thickness trough at the junction of the lamina and the lateral mass. At this point, if laminar shingling at the cranial level is severe enough to prohibit adequate laminar mobilization, you have the option of performing a partial dome or full formal laminectomy at the level above to allow more room for the caudal lamina to hinge open freely. This will also help prevent impingement of the lamina postoperatively when the neck is hyperextended. Once the trough has been drilled, the underlying soft tissue attachments are released with the use of a nerve hook and a 2 mm Kerrison rongeur. Attention is then turned to the contralateral side with the goal of creating a partial thickness trough to allow for the creation of a greenstick fracture, which serves as the laminar hinge. Our preferred method involves the use of the side-cutting burr to thin the junction between the lamina and the lateral mass using a circular motion. The mobility of the lamina is intermittently interrogated at with the use of a nerve hook until it can be freely elevated to fit the desired graft size, typically 10 mm for males and 8 mm for females.

Once all lamina have been mobilized, you can proceed with grafting and fixation. Graft trials are used to size the open edge of the laminoplasty. An appropriately fitting trial should fit securely in place and the spinal cord should be visibly decompressed. Allograft struts are then placed and secured with your fixation system of choice. We prefer the use of a plate system that bridges the lamina and the lateral mass coupled with prefabricated allograft bone implants (Figs. 4.1A and B). While some surgeons forgo grafting and rely on the plate alone for fixation, we feel that the addition of the structural graft adds stability and potentially decreasing the rate of hinge failure. Prior to inserting the graft into the patient, we recommend pretapping them by placing and removing the self-tapping screw through the graft on the back table. This minimizes the torque on the graft when the time comes to secure it in place. Once the graft is in position, carefully insert the plate, aligning the central hole over the graft. While holding the graft steady with a small straight clamp, partially insert the screw to provisionally secure the graft to the plate. At this point, you may proceed to fix the plate to the lamina and lateral mass using a drill with a depth stop. Start by drilling

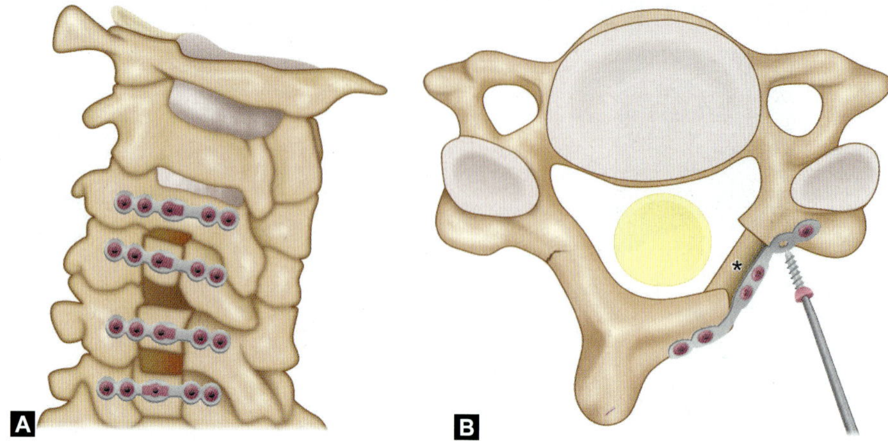

Figs. 4.1A and B: Artist's representation of our preferred laminoplasty technique using a prefabricated allograft strut (* in B) and plate fixation. Both posterior (A) and axial (B) views are shown.

and placing a single laminar screw, leaving it prod enough to provide some play in the plate. Next, ensure the lateral edge of the plate is positioned over the center of the lateral mass. This step often requires additional dissection out over the lateral masses, but again you must be careful not to disrupt the facet capsules. Once the plate is appropriately positioned you may drill and place your screws in the lateral mass before returning to complete the laminar sided fixation and final tighten the initial laminar screw. Finally, definitively tighten the graft screw, again stabilizing the graft with a small straight clamp. Final radiographs are obtained in the operating room with careful attention paid to the positioning of the lateral mass screws to ensure they do not violate the facet joints.

A layered closure is performed with the surgeon's choice of an absorbable or nonabsorbable suture for the ligamentum nuchae followed by an absorbable braided suture for the dermal layer and then an absorbable monofilament or nylon suture for the skin. Prior to closure, a subfascial posterior drain may be placed to prevent the formation of a postoperative hematoma. A soft collar may be used for comfort for the first 2 weeks postoperatively, but no range of motion (ROM) restrictions is necessary.

OUTCOMES

Patients with clinical symptoms of myelopathy can expect that laminoplasty will arrest neurologic deterioration and prevent further disability. Patients require little to no postoperative immobilization, with the collar serving the purpose of comfort and soft tissue rest. By definition, there is no concern for pseudoarthrosis with this procedure and adjacent level disease should be minimized through motion preservation.[4]

Predictors of moderate-to-severe neck pain at 2-year follow-up include the presence of anterolisthesis, an active smoking history, moderate-to-severe baseline neck pain, and lower SF-36 Mental Component Summary Scores.[5]

Compared with posterior laminectomy and fusion, laminoplasty avoids all fusion-related complications and offers potentially shorter operative time, decreased blood loss, faster recovery, decreased implant costs, decreased inpatient stay costs, and similar rates of neurologic recovery.[6-9] Several studies have also demonstrated a decreased rate of postoperative C5 palsy, as much as 25% less, in some studies. In a direct comparison, patients who had laminectomy with fusion and who sustained C5 nerve palsy had increased grade of motor weakness, increased incidence of additional nerve root involvement, and longer recovery time.[10]

A long-term follow-up of 10 years following cervical laminoplasty for myelopathy secondary to cervical spondylosis or ossification of the posterior longitudinal ligament has been described. Of the 126 patients available for follow-up, 55% maintained improved Japanese Orthopaedic Association scores; 25% of patients had decreased postoperative cervical ROM and eight patients developed increased kyphosis, which was a predictor of poor recovery.[11]

COMPLICATIONS

There are several disadvantages of laminoplasty when compared with other surgical approaches. When compared to anterior surgery, the posterior laminoplasty incision is less cosmetically appealing given the longitudinal nature and more prone to wound complications. Laminoplasty is also not expected to improve neck pain, and in some cases can exacerbate the existing neck pain. Compared with anterior fusion, laminoplasty had increased rates of nuchal pain, shoulder pain, and shoulder muscle spasm; all of which have been collectively referred to as postoperative axial symptoms.[12] The axial neck pain is one of the most notorious complications of cervical laminoplasty being reported up to 60–80% of patients, and its presence preoperatively often is an indication to consider laminectomy and fusion. However, there are several proposed strategies for decreasing the rates of axial neck and shoulder pain to include limiting decompression levels from C3–C6 versus C3–C7.[13] Most importantly, decreased rates of postoperative axial neck pain are achieved by restricting the indications for surgery to include: (1) compressive pathology spanning less than or equal to three levels; (2) a lack of diffuse axial neck pain as a predominant or significant complaint; and (3) upright lateral radiographs revealing a neutral to lordotic C2-7 sagittal angle.[14]

CASE PRESENTATION

A 60-year-old male presented with a 6-month history of progressive problems with balance and upper extremity fine motor tasks. He had no complaints of neck or arm pain. The examination revealed normal neck ROM, positive Lhermitte's phenomenon, and 4-/5 strength with hand intrinsic muscle testing. He was hyperreflexic in both upper and lower extremities, had a positive Hoffman's sign bilaterally, and upgoing toes on Babinski. He was unable to perform tandem gait without losing his balance. Plain film radiographs of the cervical spine demonstrated diffuse spondylosis with preservation of adequate cervical ROM and lordosis (Fig. 4.2). A MRI demonstrated severe spinal cord compression from C4-6 with significant myelomalacial changes most notable at the C5 level (Fig. 4.3).

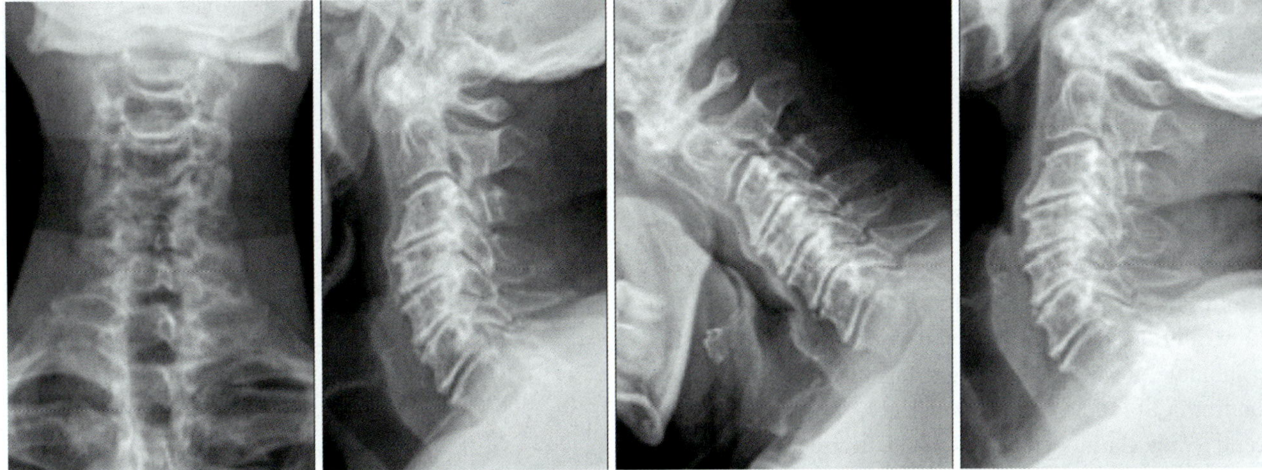

Fig. 4.2: Preoperative AP, lateral, flexion, and extension radiographs (left to right) of the cervical spine demonstrating multilevel cervical spondylosis with overall preservation of cervical range of motion and lordosis (AP: anteroposterior).

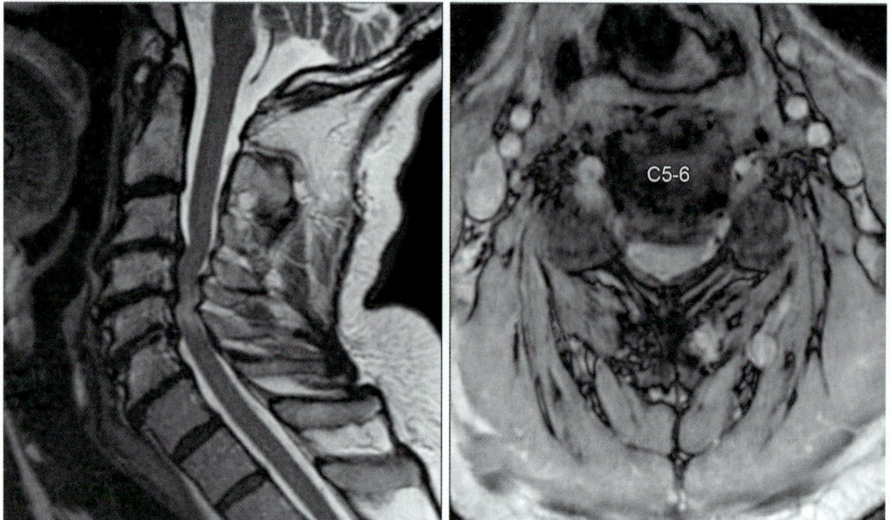

Fig. 4.3: Sagittal and axial T2 MRI scans of the cervical spine demonstrating severe multilevel cervical spinal cord compression and spinal cord signal change.

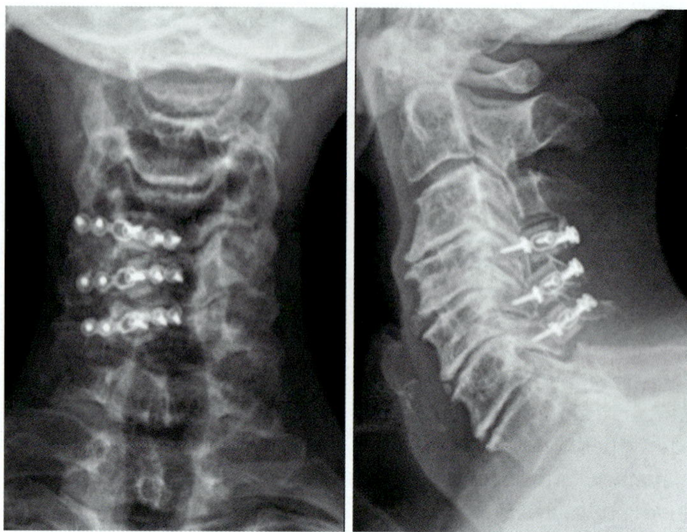

Fig. 4.4: Postoperative anteroposterior (left) and lateral (right) radiographs demonstrating a C4–6 laminoplasty. Note the partial dome laminectomy performed at C3 to prevent postoperative impingement on the C4 lamina as the cervical spine moves into extension.

The patient underwent an uncomplicated laminoplasty from C4-6. Given his significant cervical lordosis, a partial dome laminectomy was performed at C3 to prevent postoperative impingement upon the expanded C4 lamina when his neck is extended. Postoperative radiographs demonstrate well-positioned grafts and well-fixed hardware (Fig. 4.4). At the time of most recent follow-up, the patient reported no significant neck pain, subjective maintenance of his preoperative ROM, and no progression of his preoperative myelopathy symptoms.

Case Presentation

Anand Segar, Tyler Kreitz

This 72-year-old male presents with fine upper extremity motor skill dysfunction, frequent falls, and balance issues. His examination revealed weakness in both of his upper limbs, hyperreflexia, and a bilateral positive Hoffman's sign.

Preoperative X-rays show multilevel spondylosis with a well-aligned lordotic spine and no segmental instability. An MRI shows cord signal change at C3/4 with multilevel cord compression from C3/4 to C6/7. Postoperative X-rays show an open door laminoplasty at C4, 5, and 6 with a laminectomy at C3 and a partial laminectomy of the leading edge of C7 (authors preferred surgical plan) (Figs. 4.5 to 4. 9).

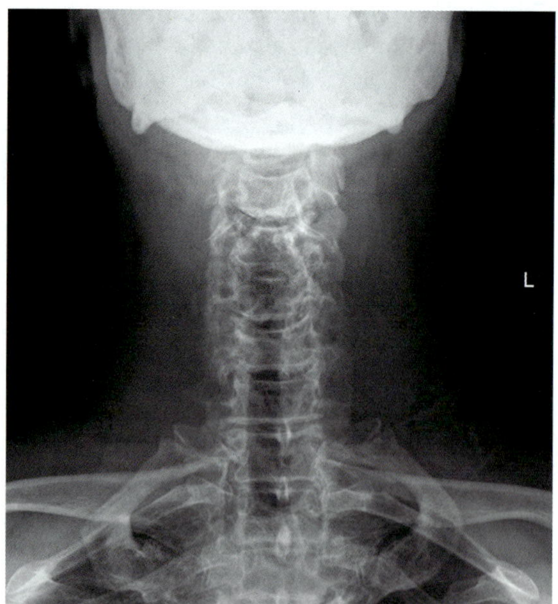

Fig. 4.5: Preoperative anteroposterior X-ray.

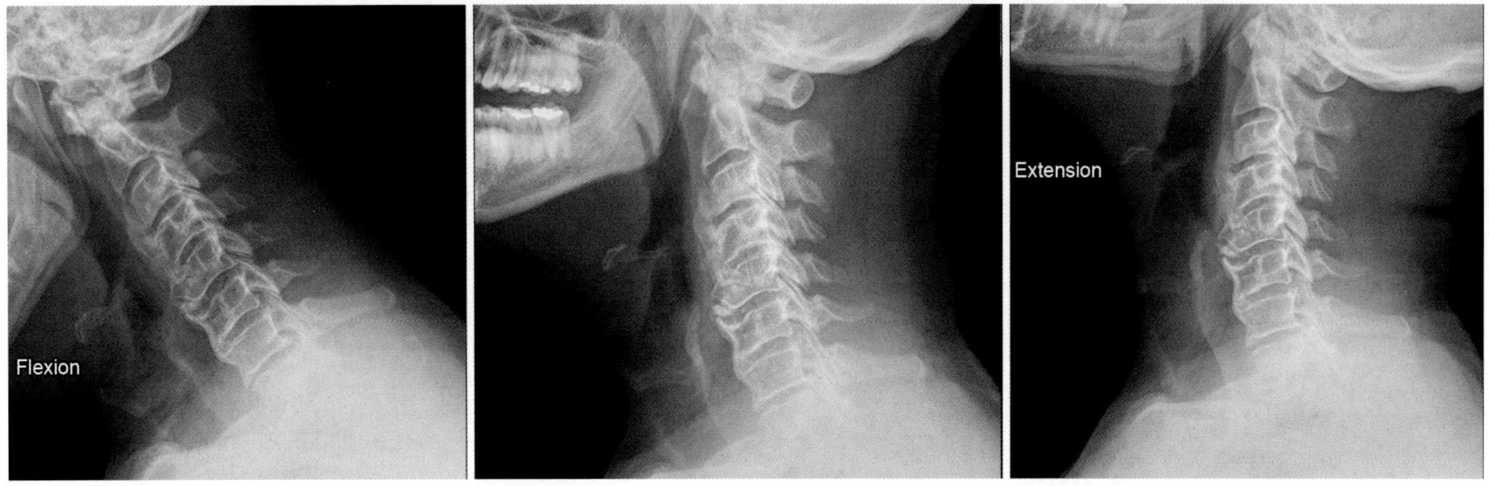

Fig. 4.6: Preoperative lateral X-rays showing spondylosis.

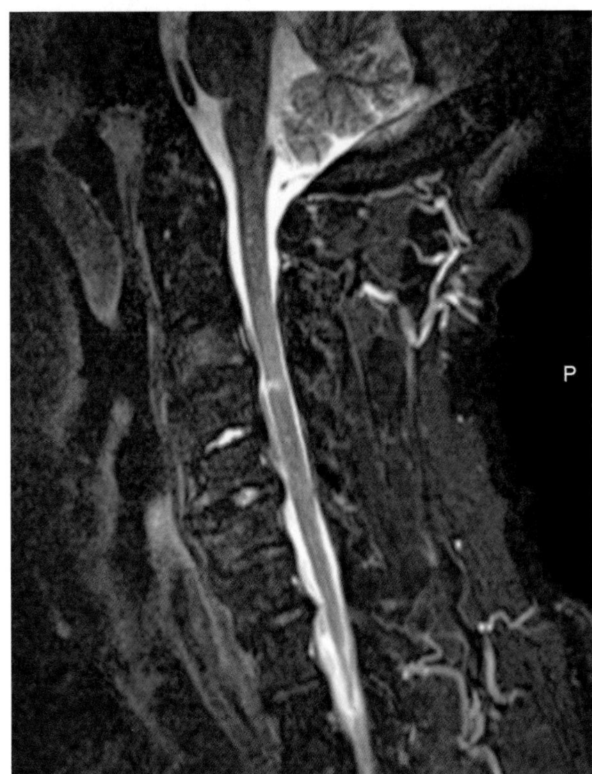

Fig. 4.7: Sagittal MRI showing compression from C3/4 to C6/7.

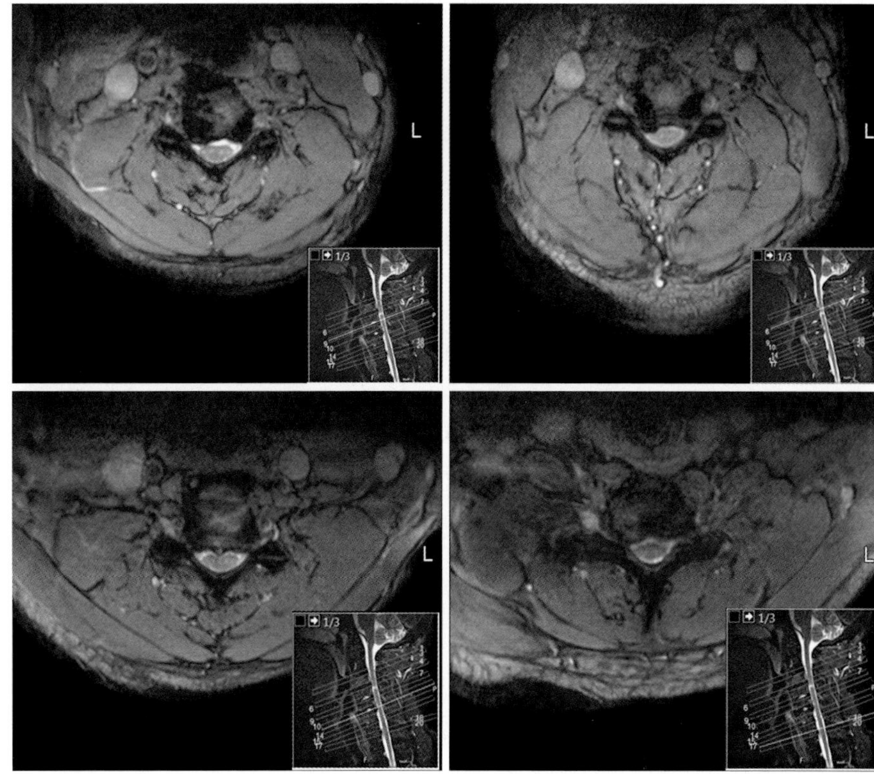

Fig. 4.8: Axial MRI images showing multilevel cord compression from C3/4 to C6/7.

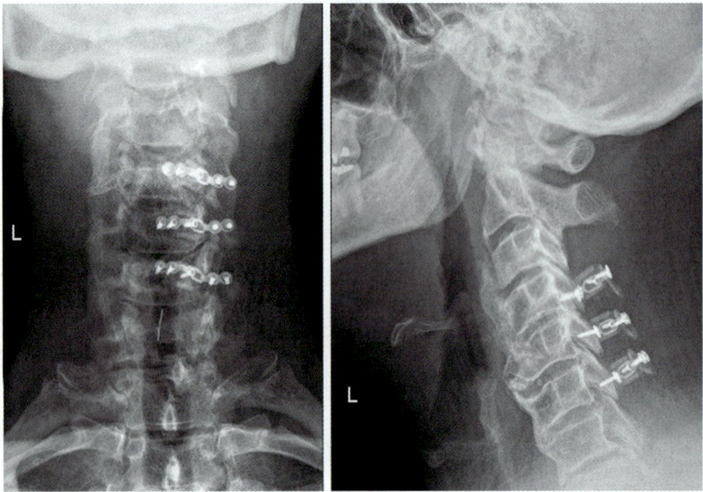

Fig. 4.9: Anteroposterior (left) and lateral (right) showing open door laminoplasty at C4–6 with a laminectomy at C3 and a partial laminectomy of the leading edge of C7.
Courtesy: Dr Alan Hilibrand.

REFERENCES

1. Panjabi WA. Clinical Biomechanics of the Spine, 2nd edition. Philadelphia, PA: Lippincott-Raven; 1990.
2. Lehman RA Jr, Taylor BA, Rhee JM, et al. Cervical laminaplasty. J Am Acad Orthop Surg. 2008;16(1):47-56.
3. Rhee JM, Daniel KRIEW. Surgical management of cervical myelopathy. J Neuro. Sci. [Turkish]. 2005;22(4):359-73.
4. Vaccaro A, Albert T. Spine Surgery: Tricks of the Trade, 3rd edition. New York, NY: Thieme Medical Publishers; 2016.
5. Kimura A, Shiraishi Y, Inoue H, et al. Predictors of persistent axial neck pain after cervical laminoplasty. Spine. 2018;43(1):10-5.
6. Heller JG, Edwards CC 2nd, Murakami H, et al. Laminoplasty versus laminectomy and fusion for multilevel cervical myelopathy: an independent matched cohort analysis. Spine.2001;26(12):1330-6.
7. Blizzard DJ, Caputo AM, Sheets CZ, et al. Laminoplasty versus laminectomy with fusion for the treatment of spondylotic cervical myelopathy: short-term follow-up. Eur Spine J. 2017;26(1):85-93.
8. Yoon ST, Hashimoto RE, Raich A, et al. Outcomes after laminoplasty compared with laminectomy and fusion in patients with cervical myelopathy: a systematic review. Spine. 2013;38(22 Suppl 1):S183-94.
9. Adogwa O, Huang K, Hazzard M, et al. Outcomes after cervical laminectomy with instrumented fusion versus expansile laminoplasty: a propensity matched study of 3185 patients. J Clin Neurosci. 2015;22(3):549-53.
10. Lee SH, Suk KS, Kang KC, et al. Outcomes and related factors of C5 palsy following cervical laminectomy with instrumented fusion compared with laminoplasty. Spine. 2016;41(10):E574-9.
11. Kawaguchi Y, Kanamori M, Ishihara H, et al. Minimum 10-year follow-up after en bloc cervical laminoplasty. Clin Orthop Relat Res. 2003;411:129-39.
12. Hosono N, Yonenobu K, Ono K. Neck and shoulder pain after laminoplasty: a noticeable complication. Spine. 1996;21(17):1969-73.
13. Hosono N, Sakaura H, Mukai Y, et al. C3-6 laminoplasty takes over C3-7 laminoplasty with significantly lower incidence of axial neck pain. Eur Spine J. 2006;15(9):1375-9.
14. Stephens BF, Rhee JM, Neustein TM, et al. Laminoplasty does not lead to worsening axial neck pain in the properly selected patient with cervical myelopathy: a comparison with laminectomy and fusion. Spine. 2017;42(24):1844-50.

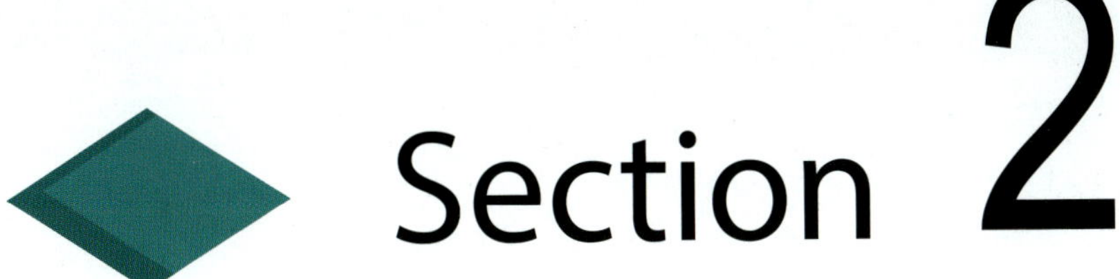

Section 2

Thoracic

- Surgical Treatment of Thoracic Disc Herniation
- Thoracic Transpedicular Decompression
- Multilevel Ponte Osteotomy for Thoracic Kyphosis
- Vertebral Column Resection

CHAPTER

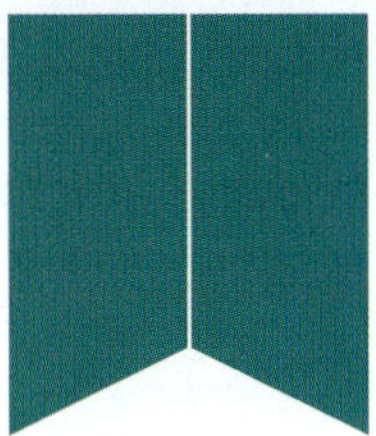

5

Surgical Treatment of Thoracic Disc Herniation

Daniel N Kiridly, Alexander Satin, David A Essig, Jeff S Silber

ANATOMY

There are 12 thoracic vertebrae in the adult spine. Each thoracic vertebra in the T2-T8 region has superior and inferior costal demi-facets in the vertebral body to articulate with the rib heads. The T10-T12 vertebrae differ in that they each have an entire costal facet in the vertebral body, whereas the T1 vertebra has an entire costal facet superiorly and a demi-facet inferiorly, and the T9 vertebra has only one demi-facet superiorly. All thoracic vertebrae, with the exception of T11 and T12, also have transverse-costal facets which articulate with the rib posteriorly. The articulations with the rib cage add significant stability to the T1-T10 vertebrae, limiting motion at these levels and making disc herniations rare. The T11 and T12 vertebrae are relatively more mobile as they articulate with the so-called "free ribs" and thus herniation is more likely at those levels.

In the thoracic spine, the facet joints are oriented vertically in the sagittal plane, which restricts flexion/extension motion in the thoracic spine, while allowing lateral bending. This is likely to prevent pathologic thoracic motion which could restrict the space required for the heart and lungs. Both the spinal cord and the spinal canal narrow in diameter in the thoracic spine, however, the size of the spinal canal decreases more dramatically in the thoracic region, resulting in the spinal cord occupying a greater portion of the canal space, making small herniations more likely to result in stenosis.[1]

The thoracic spine has an overall kyphotic alignment. Normal thoracic kyphosis increases with age and varies with gender, but generally ranges from 20° in younger individuals to 50° in older individuals.[2] Due to the kyphotic alignment of the thoracic spine, the spinal cord in this region occupies a more ventral position in the canal as it is "draped over" the anterior elements, and this is more prone to injury from disc herniation.[2]

Finally, the thoracic spinal cord is a watershed region in terms of the blood supply to the anterior spinal artery. Only a few radicular arteries supply the anterior spinal cord in the thoracic region, with the majority of the blood supply coming from the arteria radicularis magna, or the artery of Adamkiewicz. The sparse supply to the anterior spinal artery makes the thoracic spine especially prone to ischemic injury from blood supply occlusion.[3]

INDICATIONS

Thoracic disc herniation may occur asymptomatically. The true incidence of asymptomatic thoracic herniated nucleus pulposus (HNP) is not well-characterized due to a paucity of literature on the subject; however, the available literature suggests the rates are high, somewhere between 15% and 37%.[4,5] In a large series of thoracic HNPs which were operatively treated, pain (radicular, localized, or axial) was the most common symptom presenting in 76% of patients, whereas weakness and/or sensory deficits were each present in 61%, hyperreflexia/spasticity was present in 58%, and bladder deficits were present in 24%.[6] A number of studies have reported on thoracic HNP presenting with unusual symptoms including abdominal pain,[7] nausea/vomiting,[8] and flank pain,[9] suggesting a high index of suspicion is needed to make the diagnosis.

The gold standard for diagnosis of thoracic HNP is a noncontrast magnetic resonance imaging (MRI) of the thoracic spine. In patients with older metal implants which are not safe for use with MRI, a computed tomography (CT) myelogram may be used to diagnose thoracic herniations; however, in patients with significant stenosis contrast material may not flow freely, negatively impacting the image quality. Retrospective studies have been unable to differentiate radiographic qualities of asymptomatic versus symptomatic HNP, suggesting that radiographic appearance of the herniation should not be the sole criteria used to indicate operative treatment.[4]

Little characterization has been done on the natural history of symptomatic thoracic HNP owing to the rarity of the condition. One study by Brown et al.[10] found that, in a series of 55 patients with symptomatic thoracic HNP who were treated conservatively, 77% had symptomatic improvement allowing them to return to their baseline level of activity, and only 23% ended up requiring operative intervention. Moreover, studies on the outcomes of patients treated with discectomy for thoracic HNP showed that patients with severe symptoms at initial presentation had the best outcomes with operative intervention.[11] These data seem to suggest that, especially in patients who present with mild symptoms, particularly axial or radicular pain alone, conservative management plays an important role. However, for patients who present with myelopathic symptoms, in particular weakness and/or bowel or bladder dysfunction, early operative intervention is typically recommended in order to prevent the existence of persistent neurologic deficits which would significantly impact the quality of life.

TECHNIQUE

Initial efforts to treat thoracic disc herniation were done through a direct posterior approach, with extensile laminectomy and lateral retraction of the spinal cord utilizing either an extradural or intradural approach to the herniated disc. Early results of this technique showed unacceptably poor results and high complication rates, with a number of patients developing postoperative paraparesis.[12] Therefore, a number of different approaches to the thoracic disc space which minimize mobilization of the spinal cord have been developed. Each approach has a unique set of benefits and risks, making different approaches optimal for different situations in order to minimize morbidity.

For each approach, an important first step to the procedure is to correctly identify that the correct disc space is being accessed. For anterior procedures, this can be accomplished by counting the ribs under direct visualization, but for lateral and posterolateral approaches, identifying the correct level may be more challenging. Particularly for upper thoracic herniations, surrounding bony and soft tissue structures make it difficult to intraoperatively identify the correct level using lateral radiographs. Authors have proposed various potential solutions to this problem, including a CT-guided placement of a hook wire at the level of the herniation preoperatively[13] and injection of a methylene blue dye around the spinous process of interest, localized using anteroposterior (AP) radiographs.[14]

Anterior Approach: Thoracotomy

The open transthoracic approach to the thoracic spine is the most invasive and morbid of the approaches currently in use for thoracic HNP. In this approach, the patient is placed in the lateral decubitus position. Typically, a left-sided approach is utilized owing to the increased risks involved with retraction of the vena cava as compared with the thoracic aorta. Incision is carried out over the rib to be resected, typically two rib levels above the disc space of interest. The rib is dissected subperiosteally with care taken to preserve the intercostal neurovascular bundle inferior to the rib. The lung may be deflated with a double-lumen endotracheal tube if the patient can tolerate single-lung ventilation, otherwise it can be retracted laterally or superiorly. The connective tissue surrounding the remaining mediastinal structures (esophagus, aorta) must be carefully incised so they can be retracted medially, exposing the vertebral bodies. Following appropriate ligation of segmental vessels, the intercostal neurovascular bundle may be dissected to localize the foramen.

The rib head is usually resected to fully identify the pedicle. Once the correct level has been confirmed, the pedicle of the caudal vertebra for the disc space is removed to expose the spinal cord. The inferior edge of the cranial pedicle may also be partially resected to enlarge the exposure. Following this, the anterior and middle part of the disc may be removed with pituitary rongeurs. Once the disc space has been defined, a high-speed burr is utilized to create troughs in the superior and inferior vertebral bodies essentially performing a partial corpectomy. Care should be taken to thin but not violate the posterior cortex. Bony resection should be continued until the contralateral pedicle can be defined and palpated. Once bony resection is complete and the posterior cortex is thinned, a plane should be defined between the dura and the posterior cortex above and below the disc space. A combination of curettes may then be used to pull the thinned posterior cortex, posterior annulus, and posterior disc material into the defect created by the partial corpectomy. Care should be taken to ensure resection of the posterior longitudinal ligament and avoid any undue manipulation of the spinal cord. The authors prefer to perform anterior bone grafting with either iliac crest autograft or allograft followed by posterior spinal fusion with pedicle screw instrumentation across the operative disc space (Figs. 5.1A to D).

This approach provides the best visualization of and access to the disc herniation, and is particularly useful for central or paracentral herniations. In cases where extensive visualization is necessary, such as with giant herniated discs, or in which discectomy is expected to be difficult, such as with calcified discs, thoracotomy is the preferred approach. Hott et al.[15] in a series of 20 giant herniated discs treated with discectomy found the transthoracic approach to have superior short- and long-term functional outcomes to thoracoscopic and posterolateral approaches (discussed below). Moreover, the anterior approach is preferred when multiple herniations need to be addressed concurrently. Ohnishi et al.[16] had good results for 12 patients with multiple thoracic HNP treated with anterior discectomy and fusion.

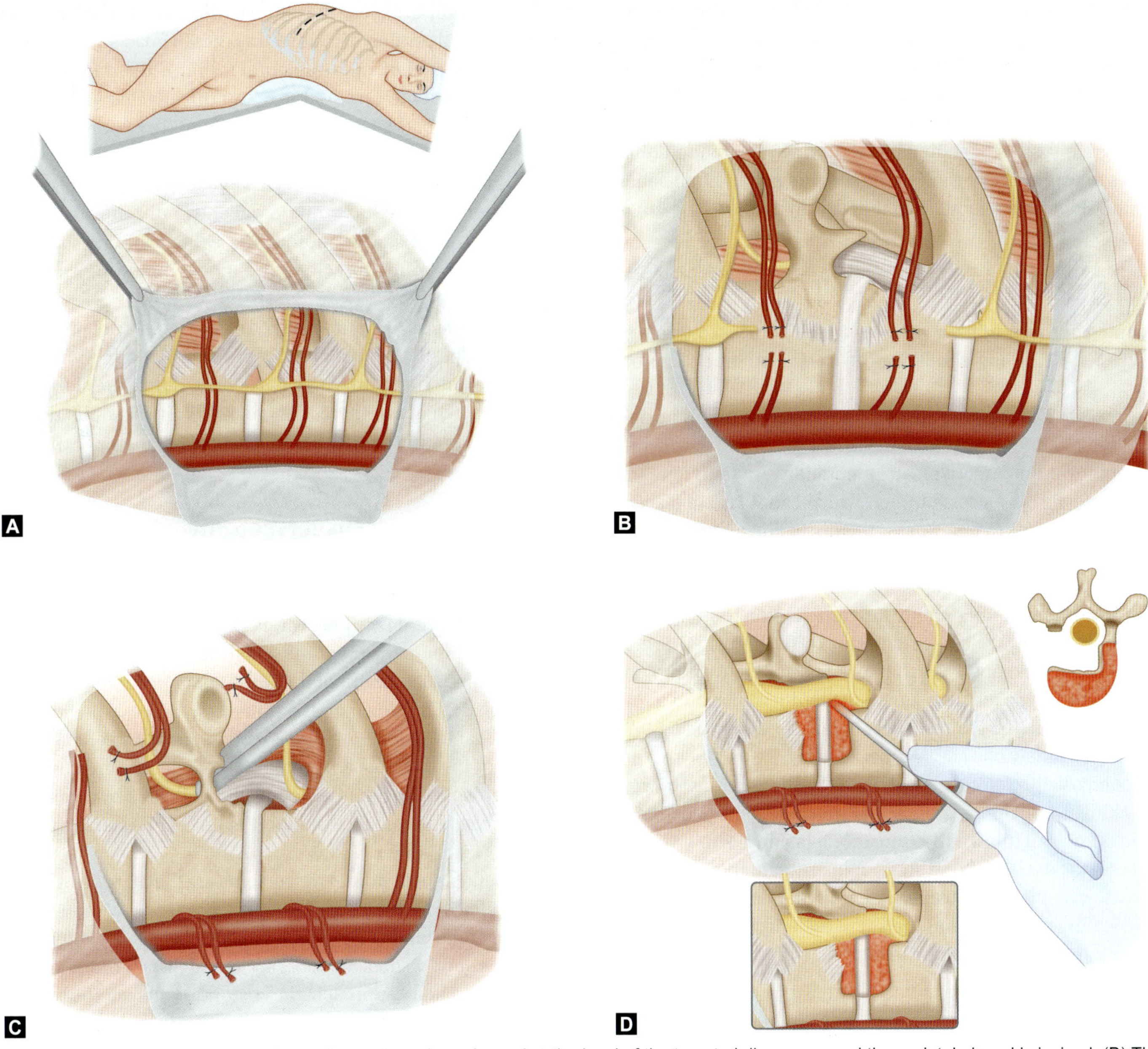

Figs. 5.1A to D: (A) Following lateral decubitus positioning, a thoracotomy is performed at the level of the targeted disc space and the parietal pleural is incised. (B) The segmental vessels are ligated, and the medial rib head (which overlies the corresponding pedicle) is excised to identify the caudal pedicle. (C) The pedicle is resected using a high-speed burr and Kerrison rongeur to identify the margins of the spinal canal and spinal cord. (D) After partial resection of the anterior disc, a partial corpectomy is performed above and below the disc space to create a cavity to pull posterior disc tissue and annulus into. This is done with a combination of reverse curettes and rongeurs. Once this is complete, the posterior longitudinal ligament is resected to complete the decompression.

Source: Bohlman HH, Thomas A. Zdeblick. Anterior excision of a thoracic discs. Bone and Joint Surg. 1988.

Unfortunately, there is significant morbidity associated with the anterior approach. Postoperative pain is usually quite significant, and intercostal neuralgia from rib resection and retraction is also difficult to manage. The need for a chest tube postoperatively is a burden to patients and may increase the length of hospital stay. There are also risks involved with retraction of mediastinal structures, including iatrogenic damage to the great vessels or esophagus requiring repair. Additionally, surgery at the lower levels may require incision of the diaphragm, and frail patients may not be able to tolerate single-lung ventilation if deflation of one of the lungs is required.

Anterior Approach: Thoracoscopic

The anterior thoracoscopic approach utilizes video-assisted thoracoscopic surgery (VATS) techniques to access the HNP in a similar way to the transthoracic approach with less morbidity.

The VATS technique involves placing the patient in the lateral decubitus position, and requires routine single-lung ventilation and deflation of the lung on the operative side in order to have room for thoracoscopic instrumentation. Three to four small incisions are made in the intercostal spaces, through which cannulas are placed to allow the endoscope and instruments to freely pass. The dissection and retraction of the mediastinal structures, as well as the general steps involved in visualizing and removing the herniated disc are essentially the same with VATS as they are with the transthoracic approach, except that thoracoscopic instrumentation is utilized.

Thoracoscopic discectomy allows excellent visualization of the herniated disc, and is particularly useful for central herniations. It also has fewer postoperative morbidities than open thoracotomy, there is typically less pain, smaller incisions, and a lower incidence of intercostal neuralgia. The rib resection is not necessary using VATS; however, a chest tube is still routinely placed postoperatively.

The video-assisted thoracoscopic surgery is not useful in all situations; however, the need for single-lung ventilation in this technique may preclude some patients from tolerating the procedure. Moreover, unlike the transthoracic approach, VATS does not provide adequate access to pass large bone grafts or instrumentation for anterior fusion, necessitating the use of endoscopic fusion systems if the spine is destabilized. Finally, endoscopic discectomy requires a unique set of technical skills associated with a significant learning curve, and surgeons not familiar with the technique may find it difficult to adopt.

Lateral Approach

The lateral extracavitary approach to the thoracic spine for HNP is a useful way to access lateral herniations with good visualization while not violating the pleural cavity. This technique is also performed in the lateral position. Dissection is taken down to approximately the medial one-fourth of the rib at the pathologic level, and carried further medially to expose the entire lamina. The rib is then dissected subperiosteally and the medial portion of it, as well as the rib head and the intercostal neurovascular bundle is resected in an extrapleural fashion. The transverse process, lamina, facet, and a portion of the vertebral body on the affected side are also resected to obtain good exposure of the lateral disc pathology. The pathologic disc is then removed in a routine fashion.

The lateral approach to thoracic HNP allows for good visualization and resection of soft lateral, as well as some paracentral disc herniations. It provides superior visualization to posterior approaches, while avoiding some of the most significant morbidities of transthoracic approaches, including single-lung ventilation and thoracotomy.

The drawbacks of this approach are that it does not provide good access to central herniations, particularly calcified central herniations. Moreover, it is difficult to repair tears in the anterior dura which may occur, due to the sharp angle that is required by this approach. Finally, there is some morbidity from the resection of the intercostal neurovascular bundle which is necessary for medial exposure when utilizing this approach.

Posterior: Costotransversectomy

The costotransversectomy is an extensive posterolateral approach to thoracic HNP which in some regards is very similar to the lateral extracavitary approach. Costotransversectomy, however, is performed with the patient prone. It involves dissection of the paraspinal musculature down to the lamina, transverse process, and most medial segment of the rib. A small portion of the medial rib is resected in an extrapleural fashion, and the transverse process, pedicle, and facet joint are also removed. Lateral subperiosteal dissection then proceeds along the pedicle and lateral body up to the disc space. The caudal pedicle can then be resected with utilization of the high-speed burr for decancellation followed by careful resection with curettes. The disc can then be accessed and is removed using reverse-angled curettes and rongeurs (Fig. 5.2).

The benefits of costotransversectomy are that it involves anatomy and an approach that should be familiar to most spine surgeons. Moreover, it involves a minimal resection of the medial rib, which results in less morbidity related to chest wall pain. It provides good visualization of soft lateral disc herniations. When compared to the lateral extracavitary approach, the costotransversectomy typically results in a shorter operative time and less blood loss, however, it has a similar complication rate.[17] The lateral extracavitary and costotransversectomy approaches are good options in the lower thoracic spine where a transthoracic approach would necessitate incision of the diaphragm.

As with the lateral extracavitary approach, the costotransversectomy is often not adequate for the treatment of central, giant, or calcified disc herniations. When

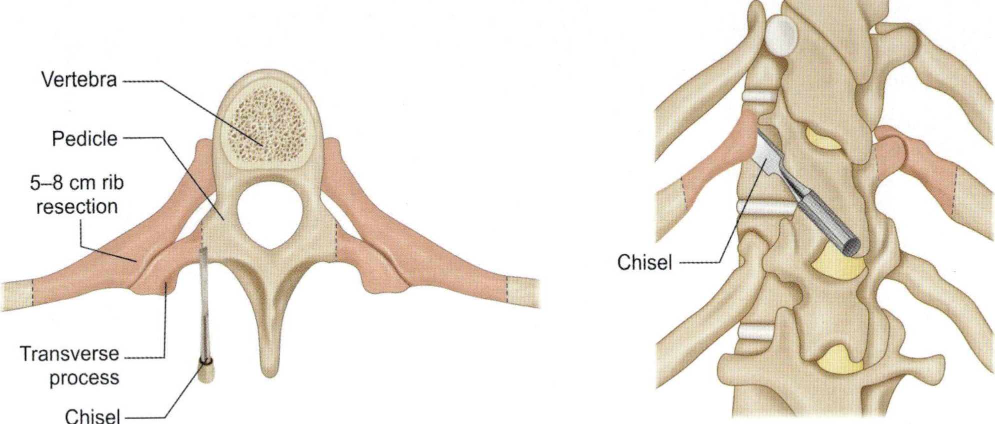

Fig. 5.2: Following exposure of the transverse process and medial rib, the transverse process is osteotomized and resected. The medial aspect of the rib is then resected after careful subperiosteal dissection and disarticulation of the costovertebral joint. This gives access to the lateral wall and disc space. Following pedicular resection, discectomy may be performed in a standard fashion. *Source:* Sundararaj GD, Venkatesh K, Babu PN, et al. Extended posterior circumferential approach to thoracic and thoracolumbar spine. Oper Orthop Traumatol. 2009;21:323-34.

compared with the other posterior approach, the transpedicular approach, the dissection around the medial rib in costotransversectomy risks pleural perforation, whereas the transpedicular approach does not.

Posterior: Transpedicular

The posterior transpedicular approach is the least-invasive of the open approaches to a thoracic disc herniation. It involves dissection only of the lateral paraspinal muscles down to the lamina, and transverse process. Then the lamina, the transverse process, and the pedicle and facet joint on the ipsilateral side of the spine are removed gaining access to the far lateral portion of the intervertebral disc. Through the pedicle, the disc space is accessed. The herniated disc is then pulled posterolaterally away from the spinal cord using reverse-angled curettes. The disc material is then resected using reverse-angled pituitary rongeurs (Fig. 5.3).

The posterior transpedicular approach involves the least surgical morbidity of any other approach to the thoracic intervertebral disc. Blood loss and operative time for this approach are also significantly less. This technique also utilizes an approach and anatomy which is familiar to spine surgeons.

Conversely, the transpedicular approach provides the poorest visualization of the medial portion of the intervertebral disc, making it a suboptimal option for central or even paracentral disc herniations. Additionally, this poor visualization makes it nearly impossible to address anterior dural tears which may occur during discectomy using this technique. It is also difficult to remove a calcified disc using this technique because it involves angled instrumentation without the ability to manipulate the disc in a more forceful manner.

Alternative, minimally-invasive approaches to thoracic disc herniations have been described in the literature but will not be extensively detailed here. One is an endoscopic posterolateral approach, which utilizes tubular retractors to perform a lateral transpedicular approach utilizing a small incision with minimal small tissue trauma. Lidar et al. described this technique and had no major complications in a series of 10 patients treated with it.[18] Another minimally invasive approach is the posterior transdural technique. In this approach, a partial unilateral laminectomy, partial facetectomy, and partial pedicle removal are performed to get down to the dura, and then a durotomy is created and the spinal cord is freed and pulled posterolaterally with a stay suture, gaining access to the disc space. This technique involves minimal bony resection, but is not appropriate for larger or central herniations, and requires the patient to be on bed rest for a period of time following surgery.[19]

OUTCOMES

Owing to the rarity of thoracic herniated discs that necessitate surgical intervention, as well as the relatively recent move away from the use of laminectomy alone to perform thoracic discectomies, there is a relative paucity of literature evaluating outcomes of different approaches to thoracic HNPs. The literature that exists tends to consist of smaller case series and retrospective cohort studies by and large. Most studies show good outcomes for each of the approaches studied; however, it is worth noting that due to the lack of prospective randomized trials, comparisons between techniques are difficult to make, and the literature may reflect results from surgeons tailoring the approach to the type of herniation identified.

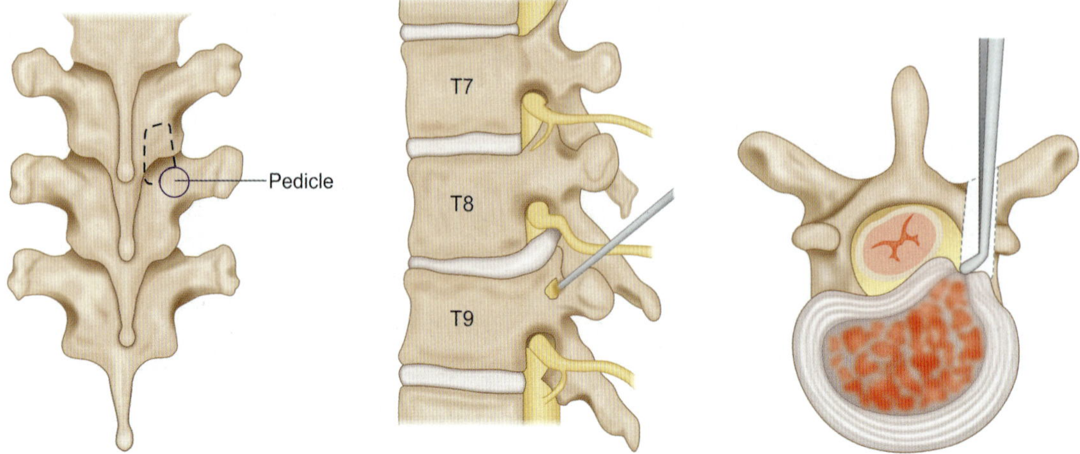

Fig. 5.3: Following identification of the anatomic landmarks for the caudal pedicle, which lies just below the targeted disc space, a facetectomy is performed followed by resection of the pedicle on the affected side. Angled curettes and rongeurs are utilized to remove the herniated disc material posterolaterally.
Source: Bilsky MH. Transpedicular approach for thoracic disc herniations. Neurosurg Focus. 2000;9(4):e3.

Anterior Approach: Thoracotomy

One of the first reports of anterior decompression of thoracic HNP was by Bohlman and Zdeblick in 1988, who examined a series of 22 thoracic herniations which were treated through either the anterior transthoracic or a costotransversectomy approach. They found 16 of the 19 patients studied had good or excellent clinical results, with 12 of the 14 patients who presented with neurologic deficits improving in motor function.[20] Hott et al. reported the outcomes of 140 patients with thoracic herniated discs with a median of 2.6 years of clinical follow-up. Most patients were treated for giant disc herniations (16 of 20) utilizing either an open anterior approach or a thoracoscopic approach, and over 90% of those patients either improved neurologically or did not have any progression. Additionally, they found that patients who underwent open thoracotomy for giant HNPs had better short- and long-term functional outcomes than those who had thoracoscopic surgery.[15] Ohnishi et al. reported outcomes on a series of 12 patients who had multiple thoracic HNPs treated with anterior discectomy and fusion. 3 of the 12 patients improved neurologically, with all patients experiencing a significant improvement in their Japanese Orthopedic Association scores for thoracic myelopathy.[16]

Anterior Approach: Thoracoscopic

Anand and Regan[11] reported one of the largest case series on thoracoscopically treated disc herniations, gathering long-term clinical data on 100 consecutive patients treated with discectomy with or without fusion, with an average follow-up of 4 years. They had a clinically successful outcome in 73% of patients at a 2-year follow-up which they defined as a 20% decrease in Oswestry Disability Index scores. They found that patients who had worse symptoms prior to treatment (in particular, patients who had symptoms other than axial back pain) tended to have greater satisfaction rates and better outcomes.[11] Quint et al. in 2012 reported outcomes for a large series of patients with thoracic disc herniations treated with thoracoscopic microdiscectomy without anterior spinal fusion. They studied 167 consecutive patients and found excellent or good outcomes in terms of pain scores and muscle strength in 79 and 80% of patients, respectively.[21]

Lateral Approach

Maiman et al. published one of the initial case series on thoracic disc herniation treated through the lateral extracavitary approach in 1984. The study included 23 patients with thoracic HNPs, 11 of which were calcified. 17 of the 23 patients had significant improvement in pain scores postoperatively, whereas 20 of the 23 patients had neurologic improvements with surgery, and no patients experienced neurologic decline.[22] Delfini et al. in 1996 presented on a series of 20 patients treated for thoracic HNP using the lateral extracavitary approach, and 15 of the patients were noted to have significant neurologic improvement at final follow-up, with follow-up periods ranging from 1 year to 8 years.[23]

Posterior: Costotransversectomy

Simpson et al. reported on a series of 21 patients with thoracic disc herniations treated via the posterolateral approach utilizing either a transpedicular approach or a costotransversectomy. They found 16 patients to have good or excellent clinical outcomes at an average of 58.3 months of follow-up, with all patients who had preoperative lower extremity weakness.[24] Lubelski et al. did a retrospective cohort analysis of 54 lateral extracavitary and costotransversectomy approaches done for all indications (not just thoracic HNP), and found that the costotransversectomy approach was associated with decreased blood loss and shorter hospital length of stay.[25]

Posterior: Transpedicular

Studies have shown generally favorable results for HNPs treated through the transpedicular approach; however, care should be taken when selecting this approach as certain disc herniations may not be amenable to successful removal with a transpedicular exposure. Levi et al. presented a series of 35 patients with thoracic disc herniations treated using the transpedicular approach, with 26 of the patients having good or fair clinical outcomes.[26] In another case series, Bilsky et al. treated 20 patients through the transpedicular approach, and had excellent results with all nonambulatory patients regaining ambulatory status. In addition, 86% of patients regained bladder function and 67% of patients had an improvement in radicular pain.[27]

Comparative Studies

There have been only a few studies comparing the outcomes of thoracic disc herniations treated using different approaches, and there have been no prospective randomized controlled trials comparing surgical approaches. Yoshihara and Yoneoka in a retrospective database study of over 25,000 patients compared in-hospital complication rates for anterior versus nonanterior approaches for thoracic disc herniation. They found higher rates of in-hospital complications, higher mortality, longer hospital stays, and higher hospital costs associated with anterior procedures.[28] Arts and Bartels in a prospective cohort study in 2014 compared 56 patients treated with mini-transthoracic anterior discectomies to 44 patients treated with transpedicular discectomies. They found no difference between the groups in terms of long-term patient-reported outcomes, and improvement in spinal cord function. However, they found that with the anterior approach, there was greater blood loss, longer hospital stays, and a higher complication rate.[29] Khoo et al. retrospectively compared patients treated with a transthoracic approach to patients treated with an endoscopic posterior transpedicular approach. They found equivalent outcomes on follow-up MRIs done at 1 year postoperatively, and noted no difference in terms of neurologic and functional outcomes.[30]

COMPLICATIONS

One of the most devastating and feared complications of thoracic discectomy is further spinal cord injury causing worsening neurologic deficits. The high incidence of this complication is what led to the abandonment of laminectomy to treat thoracic disc herniations.[12] Excessive manipulation of or pressure on the spinal cord during surgery can cause this complication. In addition to being mindful of spinal cord manipulation, it is also important to avoid inadvertent injuries to the nerve roots during the approach as this can cause tethering and traction on the spinal cord. Another serious complication of thoracic discectomy is incomplete removal of the herniated disc leading to unresolved symptoms possibly necessitating a repeat operation. This occurs in the setting of incomplete exposure and identification of relevant anatomy. The authors stress that these complications occur frequently in the setting of managing large central disc herniations or calcified discs through a posterior approach. If there is concern for these types of more complex disc herniations, strong consideration should be given to obtaining a preoperative CT scan to identify the calcified nature of the disk and approach a disc anteriorly. Many surgeons have abandoned the need for a CT and attendant radiation exposure as calcification often can be identified through the signal void seen on a T2-weighted MR image. The importance of choosing the best approach for a given thoracic disc herniation cannot be overstressed as this procedure carries a significant risk of catastrophic neurologic injury.

Instability of the spinal column postoperatively is another potential complication. This is more likely to occur with anterior decompressions, when multiple levels are addressed at the same time, or if the patient has a preexisting problem with alignment or stability. If it is suspected that discectomy may lead to excessive thoracic instability, the surgeon can address this by fusing the affected levels at the time of discectomy.

Besides the usual surgical complications of wound infection, excessive blood loss, and anesthesia risks, among others, there are risks inherent to the anterior transthoracic approach which are unique. In particular, risks related to violation of the pleural cavity include pneumonia, pleural effusion, and intercostal neuralgia. Moreover, when the great vessels are mobilized and retracted to access the posterior vertebral bodies, there is a not insignificant risk of damage to the vessels necessitating repair to prevent exsanguination.

CASE PRESENTATION

A 75-year-old woman with a past medical history of hypertension, rheumatoid arthritis, and shingles, presented to the office with acute on chronic back pain and weakness. She was being treated for lumbar spinal stenosis for years with epidural steroid injections, but over the past 2 weeks her chronic back pain became increasingly worse. This was associated with weakness and numbness in the right leg causing her to have difficulty with ambulation, and requiring her to walk with a walker. She did not complain of any bowel or bladder dysfunction at that time. On physical examination, she was noted to have marked weakness in the right lower extremity with a foot drop and decreased sensation. The remainder of her neurologic examination was normal.

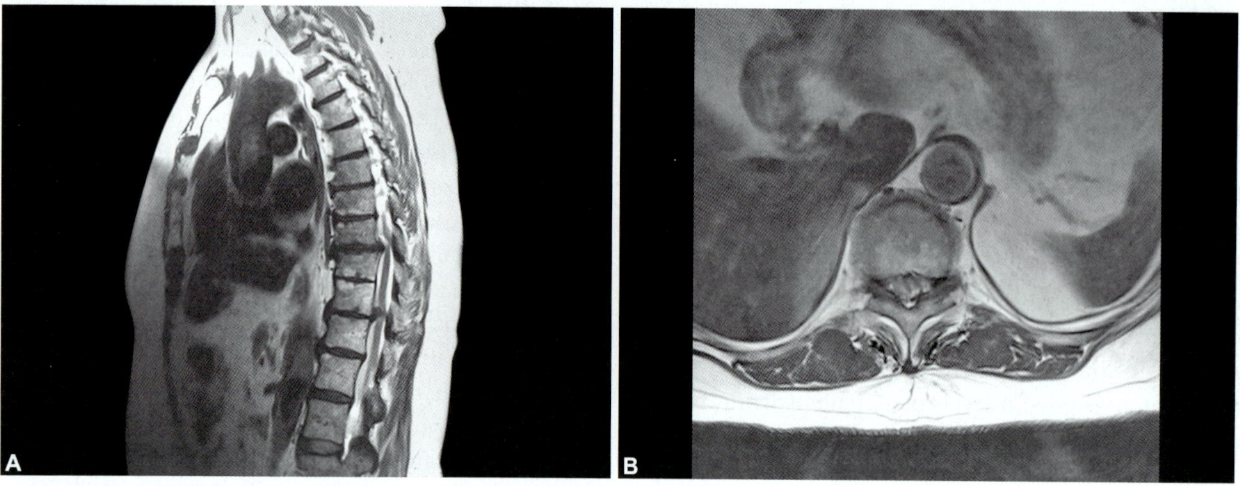

Figs. 5.4A and B: (A) Preoperative sagittal T2-weighed MRI showing the new T10-11 herniation, and the old T8-T9 herniation. (B) Preoperative axial T2-weighed MRI at the T10-11 disc level showing the extruded disc fragment causing cord compression.

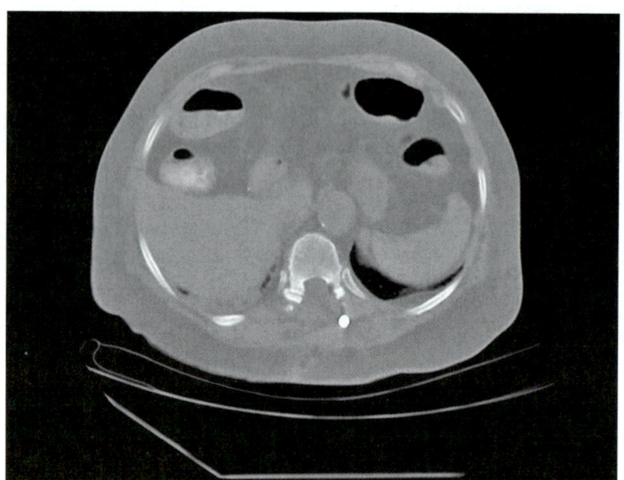

Fig. 5.5: Postoperative CT at the T10-11 level showing unilateral instrumentation, and the bony defect resulting from the transpedicular approach.

Magnetic resonance imaging showed a new central and paracentral disc herniation at T10-11 causing cord compression and cord signal changes, as well as severe degenerative change in the lumbar spine causing moderate-to-severe stenosis from L2-L5, with a grade 1 anterolisthesis of L4 on L5. In addition to these findings, the patients were also noted to have an T8–9 disc herniation that caused mild cord effacement, but had been present on imaging prior to her symptoms a year ago (Figs. 5.4A and B).

A T8 through –T12 laminectomy was performed with posterior instrumented fusion. The T10-11 disc was removed using a transpedicular approach (Fig. 5.5). She also underwent an L2-L5 laminectomy and L4-5 posterior instrumented fusion during that operation. She tolerated the surgery without complication, and was discharged to a rehab facility postoperatively. Her strength in the right leg gradually improved to the point where she could stand on her own and ambulate with assistance, and her sensory deficits and back pain improved significantly.

REFERENCES

1. Lee RA, van Zundert AA, Breedveld P, et al. The anatomy of the thoracic spinal canal investigated with magnetic resonance imaging (MRI). Acta Anaesthesiol Belg. 2007;58(3):163-7.
2. Fon GT, Pitt MJ, Thies AC Jr. Thoracic kyphosis: range in normal subjects. AJR Am J Roentgenol. 1980;134(5):979-83.
3. Shamji MF, Maziak DE, Shamji FM, et al. Circulation of the spinal cord: an important consideration for thoracic surgeons. Ann Thorac Surg. 2003;76(1):315-21.
4. Awwad EE, Martin DS, Smith KR Jr, et al. Asymptomatic versus symptomatic herniated thoracic discs: their frequency and characteristics as detected by computed tomography after myelography. Neurosurg. 1991;28(2):180-6.
5. Wood KB, Blair JM, Aepple DM, et al. The natural history of asymptomatic thoracic disc herniations. Spine (Phila Pa 1976). 1997;22(5):525-9.
6. Stillerman CB, Chen TC, Couldwell WT, et al. Experience in the surgical management of 82 symptomatic herniated thoracic discs and review of the literature. J Neurosurg. 1998;88(4):623-33.
7. Chirchiglia D, Della Torre A, Stroscio CA, et al. Intervertebral thoracic herniation disc presenting as acute abdomen. J Neurosurg Sci. 2018;62(4):522-3.

8. Rohde RS, Kang JD. Thoracic disc herniation presenting with chronic nausea and abdominal pain. A case report. J Bone Joint Surg Am. 2004;86-A(2):379-81.
9. Ozturk C, Tezer M, Sirvanci M, et al. Far lateral thoracic disc herniation presenting with flank pain. Spine J. 2006;6(2):201-3.
10. Brown CW, Deffer PA Jr, Akmakjian J, et al. The natural history of thoracic disc herniation. Spine (Phila Pa 1976). 1992;17(6 Suppl):S97-102.
11. Anand N, Regan JJ. Video-assisted thoracoscopic surgery for thoracic disc disease: Classification and outcome study of 100 consecutive cases with a 2-year minimum follow-up period. Spine (Phila Pa 1976). 2002;27(8):871-9.
12. Logue V. Thoracic intervertebral disc prolapse with spinal cord compression. J Neurol Neurosurg Psychiatr. 1952;15(4):227-41.
13. Sammon PM, Gibson R, Fouyas I, et al. Intraoperative localisation of spinal level using preoperative CT-guided placement of a flexible hook-wire marker. Br J Neurosurg. 2011;25(6):778-9.
14. Paolini S, Ciappetta P, Missori P, et al. Spinous process marking: a reliable method for preoperative surface localization of intradural lesions of the high thoracic spine. Br J Neurosurg. 2005;19(1):74-6.
15. Hott JS, Feiz-Erfan I, Kenny K, et al. Surgical management of giant herniated thoracic discs: analysis of 20 cases. J Neurosurg Spine. 2005;3(3):191-7.
16. Ohnishi K, Miyamoto K, Kanamori Y, et al. Anterior decompression and fusion for multiple thoracic disc herniation. J Bone Joint Surg Br. 2005;87(3):356-60.
17. Lubelski D, Abdullah KG, Steinmetz MP, et al. Lateral extracavitary, costotransversectomy, and transthoracic thoracotomy approaches to the thoracic spine: review of techniques and complications. J Spinal Disord Tech. 2013;26(4):222-32.
18. Lidar Z, Lifshutz J, Bhattacharjee S, et al. Minimally invasive, extracavitary approach for thoracic disc herniation: technical report and preliminary results. Spine J. 2006;6(2): 157-63.
19. Coppes MH, Bakker NA, Metzemaekers JD, et al. Posterior transdural discectomy: a new approach for the removal of a central thoracic disc herniation. Eur Spine J. 2012;21(4): 623-8.
20. Bohlman HH, Zdeblick TA. Anterior excision of herniated thoracic discs. J Bone Joint Surg Am. 1988;70(7):1038-47.
21. Quint U, Bordon G, Preissl I, et al. Thoracoscopic treatment for single level symptomatic thoracic disc herniation: a prospective followed cohort study in a group of 167 consecutive cases. Eur Spine J. 2012;21(4):637-45.
22. Maiman DJ, Larson SJ, Luck E, et al. Lateral extracavitary approach to the spine for thoracic disc herniation: report of 23 cases. Neurosurg. 1984;14(2):178-82.
23. Delfini R, Di Lorenzo N, Ciappetta P, et al. Surgical treatment of thoracic disc herniation: a reappraisal of Larson's lateral extracavitary approach. Surg Neurol. 1996;45(6):517-22; discussion 522-3.
24. Simpson JM, Silveri CP, Simeone FA, et al. Thoracic disc herniation. Re-evaluation of the posterior approach using a modified costotransversectomy. Spine (Phila Pa 1976). 1993;18(13):1872-7.
25. Lubelski D, Abdullah KG, Mroz TE, et al. Lateral extracavitary vs. costotransversectomy approaches to the thoracic spine: reflections on lessons learned. Neurosurg. 2012;71(6): 1096-102.
26. Levi N, Gjerris F, Dons K. Thoracic disc herniation. Unilateral transpedicular approach in 35 consecutive patients. J Neurosurg Sci. 1999;43(1):37-42; discussion 42-3.
27. Bilsky MH. Transpedicular approach for thoracic disc herniations. Neurosurg Focus. 2000;9(4):e3.
28. Yoshihara H, Yoneoka D. Comparison of in-hospital morbidity and mortality rates between anterior and nonanterior approach procedures for thoracic disc herniation. Spine (Phila Pa 1976). 2014;39(12):E728-33.
29. Arts MP, Bartels RH. Anterior or posterior approach of thoracic disc herniation? A comparative cohort of mini-transthoracic versus transpedicular discectomies. Spine J. 2014;14(8):1654-62.
30. Khoo LT, Smith ZA, Asgarzadie F, et al. Minimally invasive extracavitary approach for thoracic discectomy and interbody fusion: 1-year clinical and radiographic outcomes in 13 patients compared with a cohort of traditional anterior transthoracic approaches. J Neurosurg Spine. 2011;14(2):250-60.

CHAPTER

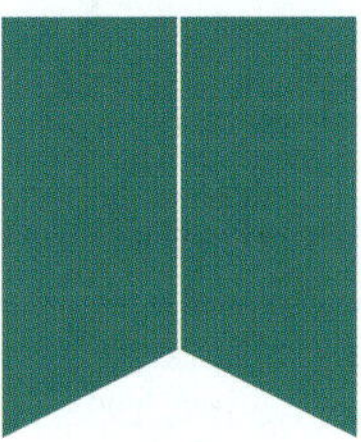

6

Thoracic Transpedicular Decompression

Alexander M Satin, Daniel N Kiridly, David A Essig, Jeff S Silber

ANATOMY

The thoracic spine is a unique structure that consists of 12 vertebrae. This is in contrast to the cervical and lumbar spines, which consists of seven and five vertebrae, respectively. The overall alignment of the thoracic spine is kyphotic, while the adjacent cervical and lumbar spines have a lordotic alignment. The amount of thoracic kyphosis varies with age and gender, but averages 20° in younger patients and 50° in older patients.[1] The kyphosis of the thoracic spine is due to the unique structure of the vertebral bodies. The anterior portion of the vertebral bodies is 2–3 mm shorter than the posterior portion.[2]

The unique and variable orientation of the thoracic spine articulations are essential to the motion and injury patterns encountered in the thoracic spine. In the proximal thoracic spine, the facet joints are coronally oriented. As a result, the proximal segment is able to resist anterior translational forces. However, there is little resistance to rotational forces at these levels. In the lower thoracic spine, the facet joints change to a sagittal orientation. As a result, these levels have a greater resistance to rotational forces. Motion in the thoracic spine is also limited by its articulations with the rib cage. This endows the thoracic spine with a higher energy threshold for injury than the adjacent cervical and lumbar spines.[3] However, this rigidity increases the incidence of fracture in the midthoracic segment when compared to the more flexible cervicothoracic and thoracolumbar junctions.

Understanding the unique pedicular anatomy of the thoracic spine is crucial for the safe placement of instrumentation and transpedicular decompression. The pedicles are generally oriented at approximately 10° in a posterolateral to anteromedial direction. In the upper thoracic spine, the pedicles are situated directly inferior to the superior articular process and at the top of transverse process. In comparison, the pedicles in the lower thoracic spine are at the level of the middle to lower half of the transverse process.[4]

INDICATIONS

The transpedicular approach provides ventrolateral exposure to the thoracic spine, and thus allows for circumferential decompression and instrumentation through a single, posterior approach. It is a versatile approach that can be modified for variety of procedures, ranging from biopsy to two column (anterior-posterior) reconstruction. Pathology of the ventral thoracic spine includes disc herniations, vertebral body pathologic fractures, spinal tuberculosis (TB), osteomyelitis/discitis, primary or secondary spinal tumors, spinal epidural abscesses, and trauma (i.e. unstable thoracic burst fractures). Patterson and Arbit described the transpedicular approach in 1978 for the treatment of protruded thoracic discs.[5]

Traditional posterior decompression offers limited ventral exposure while anterior approaches have the inherent risk of injury to the pleura and the underlying lung, mediastinum, and heart. While ventral access can be achieved posteriorly via costotransversectomy and extracavitary approaches, these approaches necessitate rib head resection and have inherent morbidity. As a result, the ability to perform a posterolateral approach through the pedicles to treat midline thoracic pathology is a valuable tool for spine surgeons. Unlike the standard transthoracic approach, the transpedicular approach does not necessitate perioperative lung collapse, and thus single-lung ventilation. Many patients, particularly patients with preexisting pulmonary dysfunction, are unable to tolerate single-lung ventilation. Furthermore, access to the upper thoracic spine through a transpedicular approach does not necessitate work around the great vessels, as is the case with ventral approaches. Patients with traumatic spinal fractures will often have multiple injuries and be unable to undergo early anterior decompression and stabilization. As a result, the posterior transpedicular approach may allow earlier decompression and stabilization in comparison to anterior procedures.

Ultimately, the surgical approach is dictated by a combination of pathology location, patient comorbidities, extent of disease, and surgeon familiarity. Nevertheless, the transpedicular approach provides an extensive exposure and can be employed in patients with primary and secondary spinal tumors with lytic destructive vertebral body lesions associated with high-grade epidural compression and/or instability. It may also be beneficial when performing an open biopsy of tumor in the ventrolateral spinal canal. A bilateral approach is necessary when performing extensive ventral debulking and/or corpectomy as a unilateral transpedicular approach does not offer adequate exposure for decompression of the medial aspects of the vertebral body.

Spinal TB frequently causes kyphotic deformity, neurologic deficit, and even paralysis. Despite extensive control efforts by the World Health Organization and local health departments, the TB epidemic persists in certain areas. Most patients with spinal TB can be cured with conservative pharmacologic treatment, but surgical methods for the treatment of spinal TB are necessary in certain cases. Although the anterior and anterolateral approaches have been traditionally preferred, they are complicated by complex anatomic layers, major vessels, and nerves. Furthermore, patient age combined with comorbid cardiovascular and respiratory disease make anterior approaches and single-lung ventilation challenging. More recent literature has demonstrated that a single-stage procedure consisting of transpedicular decompression, debridement, posterior instrumentation, and fusion is an effective and safe method in the treatment of thoracic TB with kyphosis and spinal cord compression.[6]

TECHNIQUE[7,8]

A careful review of all imaging studies prior to the operative intervention is critical. Cross-sectional imaging with three-dimensional reconstructions—magnetic resonance imaging (MRI) and computed tomography (CT) scans—allows for evaluation of pedicular anatomy, which varies throughout the thoracic spine. Patients complaining of lower extremity swelling and/or pain as well as prolonged paresis should be assessed with bilateral lower extremity venous Doppler ultrasound. Patients with a deep vein thrombosis (DVT) are then evaluated for placement of inferior vena cava filter.

Neuromonitoring with somatosensory-evoked potentials (SSEPs) and motor-evoked potentials (MEPs) are used due to the risk of neurologic injury with exposure, instrumentation, and deformity correction. A thorough discussion with the anesthesia team is critical for optimizing neural function. A clear mean arterial pressure (MAP) goal should be discussed. It is generally recommended to maintain a MAP above 85 mm Hg.

Following dual lumen general endotracheal intubation, a Foley catheter, compression boots, arterial monitoring, and venous lines are placed. A dual lumen tube is used in case single lung ventilation is needed. The patient is then placed in the prone position on a radiolucent table (Jackson) with careful padding of all bony prominences. The patient's arms are tucked at the side. The head is placed in a Mayfield head holder if fusion involving the cervicothoracic junction is planned. Fluoroscopy is used for localization and to evaluate the depth of exposure to avoid anterior breach of the vertebral body. For midthoracic interventions, anterior-posterior radiographs are obtained to count the ribs and/or pedicles. Lateral X-rays are used to localize at the cranial and caudal ends of the thoracic spine.

Antibiotics are administered prior to incision. The authors prefer weight-based dosing of cefazolin. In cases of penicillin allergic patients, weight-based vancomycin is used. In noninfection cases, the authors do not administer antibiotics beyond the first 24 hours. However, if polymethylmethacrylate (PMMA) is used as part of the reconstruction, 1 g of tobramycin is added to the PMMA in an effort to reduce infection. Surgical wounds are copiously irrigated prior to closure with antibiotic solution. Utilization of a plastic and reconstructive surgeon is assessed on a case-by-case basis. Vancomycin powder is applied to the surgical site prior to closure in cases with instrumentation and/or infection.

To control bleeding, we employ thrombotic agents such as thrombin Gelfoam® (Pharmacia & Upjohn, Kalamazoo, MI) and matrix hemostatic sealant (FloSeal®; Baxter Corp., Freemont, CA). URGICEL® Fibrillar™ (Ethicon, Somerville, NJ), an absorbable oxidized regenerated cellulose, aids in local clot formation and is helpful in achieving hemostasis. Bipolar sealers, like the Aquamantys™ (Medtronic, Dublin, Republic of Ireland), are utilized in addition to traditional electrocautery, particularly in trauma and oncologic cases. Preoperative embolization of the affected vertebra may be beneficial in limiting blood loss, especially in cases of metastatic renal cell and thyroid tumors.

A posterior midline incision is utilized for both unilateral and bilateral approaches. In cases of unilateral decompression, dissection of the ipsilateral erector spinae muscles is sufficient. The incision is centered over the pathological level(s) and extended two levels above and below if instrumentation is planned. The ligamentous attachments and paraspinal muscles are dissected to the lateral aspect of the transverse process at the levels of decompression and instrumentation.

The posterolateral decompression, including laminectomy, pediculectomy and removal of facets is performed using a 2 mm matchstick burr (M8) on the Midas Rex drill (Medtronic, Inc., Fort Worth, TX) and Kerrison rongeurs. The posterolateral decompression is continued to the adjacent laminae. The inferior aspect of the superior facet can be removed to gain access to the pedicle. If unable to locate the pedicle visually, a gearshift can be used to localize and penetrate the pedicle under biplanar fluoroscopic guidance. The gearshift should not be advanced beyond 80% of the distance to the anterior cortex.[4] The pediculectomy is started centrally with the burr followed by gradually "hollowing-out" of the pedicle via progressively larger curettes. Care should be taken to preserve the medial wall of the pedicle, as a breach can lead to neural injury, dural tear, and excessive epidural bleeding. Once the lateral aspect of the spinal canal is exposed, an angled instrument—i.e. angled curettes, Woodson dental instrument—can be used to remove the pathologic entity from the ventral thecal sac (Figs. 6.1A to D).

This approach allows for posterior vertebrectomy without having to dissect out the rib or violate the costovertebral articulation, thus reducing the risk of pleural injury. The dura can then be circumferentially visualized which allows for removal of the vertebral body using high-speed burr and/or pituitary rongeurs.

The compressive bony fragments that occur in burst fractures can be removed with angled curettes and Kerrison rongeurs. Additional fracture fragments can be impacted into the vertebral body to fill bone voids and provide support to the damaged anterior column. Care should be taken to avoid retraction of the thecal sac. In the acute trauma setting, a reduction maneuver by distraction to achieve ligamentotaxis is performed after placing pedicle screws and rods bilaterally.

In the spinal TB cases, pedicle screws are placed into the unaffected inferior and superior levels surrounding the lesion. Screws on the less affected side are fixed temporarily with a rod. Often, costotransversectomy and removal of the articular process, and pedicle are required on the most severely affected side of the lesion to

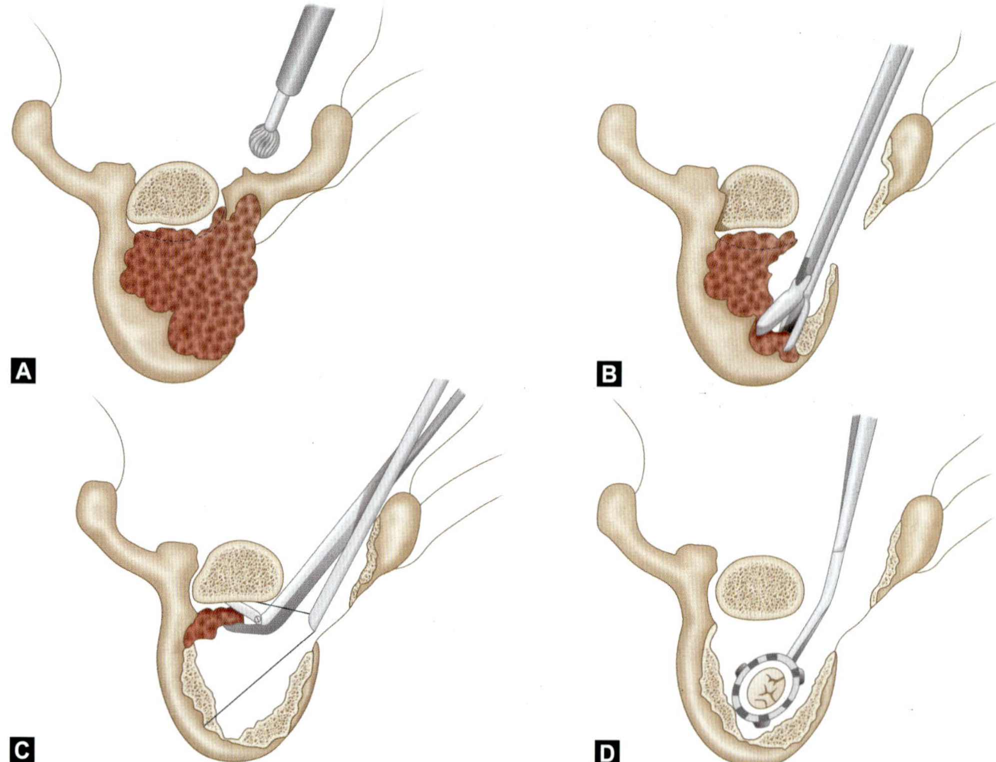

Figs. 6.1A to D: (A) Following laminectomy, a high-speed burr is utilized to perform a transpedicular resection. (B) Lateral tumor resection is performed with a combination of rongeurs and curettes. (C) A plane between the ventral dura and the epidural mass is defined and tumor abutting the cord is carefully resected. (D) Following decompression and vertebrectomy, a cage filled with bone graft is introduced into the void.

Source: Herkowitz et al. Rothman-Simeone. The Spine, 6th edition, Chapter 85, Figure 16.

drain prevertebral abscesses and expose diseased vertebral bodies. The thoracic nerve roots at the level can be sacrificed for improved exposure. Curettes are used to remove sequestra, abscesses, infected disc and endplates, caseous necrosis, and granulation tissues as thoroughly as possible. This can be performed through one or both pedicles by drill, according to the range of lesion. As a safety measure, we recommend to preserve the medial aspect of pedicles. If bilateral aspects of the vertebra are severely involved, the temporary rod is switched to the other side, and the same debridement procedure can be performed. A local antibiotic therapy with 0.75 g streptomycin and 0.3 g isoniazid are routinely used at the surgical site. Specimens should be sent for histopathologic examination and culture.[6]

In cases with epidural tumor, the authors often utilize tenotomy scissors for dissection. Bipolar cautery on a low setting is helpful to establish a plane between tumor and dura. The dissection is extended from normal dural planes and is extended around the dura. Tumor is then dissected off nervous tissue prior to ligation at cord levels when indicated. Nerve roots are only ligated if their encased in tumor and removal with maximize resection. Tumor adjacent to the lumbar nerve roots and/or plexus can be more aggressively dissected. The posterior longitudinal ligament (PLL) is cut lateral to the dura and an intralesional curettage of the vertebral body is accomplished with curettes and pituitary rongeurs. The PLL is identified at the dural margin and dissected with a Woodson instrument and tenotomy scissors to strip it from the anterior dura. Resecting the PLL provides a clean anterior margin on the dura. The adjacent disc spaces can then be freed.

Generally, two large-bore drains are left in the epidural space to prevent hematoma formation. Patients are typically transferred to the surgical intensive care unit postoperatively for appropriate resuscitation and neurologic checks. Patients are given intravenous fluid until they can tolerate oral intake. Patient-controlled analgesia is utilized and managed by anesthesia. Patients are usually transferred to the surgical floor after 24 hours. Physical and occupational therapy is started as soon as possible to mobilize the patient. A thoracolumbar spinal orthosis is applied. Pharmacologic DVT prophylaxis is utilized in select patients after discussion with collaborating providers.

OUTCOMES

Traditionally, anterior transthoracic approaches have been utilized to address various pathological entities of the ventral spine. However, due to advances in surgical technique and favorable outcomes, anterior spinal pathology is increasingly being addressed via the posterior, transpedicular approach. As such, Lu et al. sought to evaluate changes in their practice patterns and compared outcomes of thoracolumbar corpectomies performed anteriorly to those performed posteriorly via the transpedicular approach.[9] The authors retrospectively evaluated 80 patients who underwent corpectomies for a variety of pathological entities (tumor, osteomyelitis, and burst fractures); 20 anterior-only procedures, 26 anterior–posterior procedures, and 34 posterior, transpedicular procedures. In the past, the authors utilized only anterior-based approaches for thoracolumbar corpectomies. The authors compared complications, neurological outcome, morbidity, and other perioperative factors. There were no demographic differences in the surgical cohorts besides presence of metastatic disease, which was more common in the transpedicular group ($p < 0.05$). There were two perioperative deaths (sepsis and cardiac arrest) in the anterior surgery group and none in the posterior. There was no difference in operative time and estimated blood loss between the anterior-alone and posterior-alone groups ($p > 0.05$). There was no significant difference ($p = 0.63$) in complications when comparing patients who underwent anterior approaches (both anterior only and anterior–posterior) to those undergoing transpedicular approaches. However, patients in the transpedicular group had a statistically significant improvement in neurological function [American Spinal Injury Association (ASIA) score] when compared to those in the anterior surgery group ($p = 0.043$). A follow-up was longer in the anterior surgery group, and thus allowing for more time for disease recurrence and neurologic decline. However, the authors also state that the immediate circumferential decompression afforded by the transpedicular corpectomy may have increased neurologic improvement when compared to a staged procedure.

In 2016, Luo et al. shared their experience using single-stage transpedicular decompression, debridement, posterior instrumentation, and fusion in aged patients (>65 years) with thoracic TB, kyphosis, and spinal cord compression.[6] They retrospectively reported 37 cases of thoracic TB (T2-T11) with kyphosis and spinal cord compression in patients with an average age of 72.08 ± 4/49 years. No mortalities occurred during the follow-up period of 41.43 ± 3.40 months. A solid fusion was confirmed with CT in 36 of 37 cases. Patients experienced neurologic improvement at the last follow-up; 10 cases rated as ASIA classification grade D and 27 cases ASIA grade E. Preoperative examination showed an A lesion in one patient, B in five patients, C in 20 patients, and D in 11 patients. They also showed a statistically significant ($p < 0.001$) difference in postoperative Cobb angle; 39.46 ± 4.71° preoperatively and 22.32 ± 3.41° postoperatively. The authors concluded that a single-stage procedure consisting of transpedicular decompression, debridement, posterior instrumentation, and fusion is an effective and safe alternative to the extensive anterior-posterior interventions previously used to treat spinal TB in the past.

Murrey et al. retrospectively reviewed their outcomes following thoracolumbar transpedicular decompression and/or osteotomy in 59 patients; 37 deformity cases, 22 tumor or infection cases.[10] More specifically, they sought to evaluate the procedure's efficacy in achieving spinal canal decompression, spinal fusion, deformity correction, and patient outcomes. The authors utilize the term "eggshell" procedure which encompasses procedures ranging from simple transpedicular decompression and posterior fusion to more complex procedures, including transpedicular vertebrectomy and strut-grafting or pedicle subtraction (closing wedge) osteotomy with posterolateral fusion. The average follow-up was 4.5 ± 2.5 years (range 1–10 years). All patients (14) with incomplete spinal cord injuries improved. No patients worsened neurologically from the eggshell procedure alone. All patients with adequate follow-up achieved solid radiographic fusion. Patients who underwent surgery for kyphotic deformity experienced average sagittal correction of 26.2° (range 14–43°) immediately following surgery; average loss was 5.5° at follow-up (range 0–16°). The patients with more than 2-year follow-up, 92.6% were satisfied with their procedure. However, in the same group of patients, the pooled SF-36 scores were significantly lower than normal ($p < 0.001$). The authors concluded that "the transpedicular technique offers a safe and reliable way to achieve good results, including improvement in neurologic function, stabilization of the spinal column, and correction of alignment."[10]

Wong et al. described their technique and experience using a modified transpedicular approach for thoracolumbar corpectomies.[11] In cases of anterior column reconstruction via the transpedicular approach, nerve roots are often sacrificed for the passage of large constructs. However, the authors utilized bilateral expandable cages, allowing for passage of hardware with nerve root preservation—cages passed in collapsed state and subsequently expanded once in proper position. They reported on five patients, four men and one woman, who underwent their modified technique with an average follow-up of 3.3 months. Four patients had vertebral metastases and one patient have vertebral osteomyelitis and collapse. There were no perioperative complications and no nerve roots were damaged or sacrificed. Two patients who were ASIA E preoperatively remained intact after surgery. The three patients who had deficits prior to surgery all improved by 1 grade on the ASIA scale. The authors noted correction of vertebral height as well as sagittal and coronal deformity.

Danisa et al. retrospectively studied 49 consecutive nonparaplegic patients with unstable thoracolumbar burst fractures treated at their institution.[12] Their study consisted of three treatment groups—(1) 16 patients who underwent anterior decompression and instrumented fusion; (2) 27 patients who underwent posterior decompression and fusion; and (3) six patients who had combined anterior–posterior surgery. Of the 27 individuals in the posterior group, 12 were treated by direct surgical decompression via a posterolateral transpedicular approach. The remaining 15 patients underwent indirect decompression with the aid of distraction forces, attributed to the ligamentotaxis of the PLL. The groups were similar in regards to age, gender, level of injury, degree of canal compromise, neurologic impairment, and kyphosis. The patients treated via the posterior approach alone had a significant decrease in operative times ($p < 0.0003$) and blood loss ($p < 0.008$) compared to the anterior-alone and combined anterior-posterior groups. The posterior group received significantly less units of blood via transfusion than the anterior group ($p = 0.01$). Furthermore, there was no significant intergroup difference with respect to kyphotic correction, neurological function, pain assessment, or the ability to return to work. As a result, the authors concluded that the posterior-alone approach is as effective as anterior or anterior–posterior surgery when treating unstable thoracolumbar burst fractures while taking less time and causing less blood loss. In addition, posterior surgery was associated with lower costs ($p = 0.0012$). Of note, the observed cost difference could not be attributed to differences in implant costs amongst the treatment groups.

Mavrogenis et al. treated 25 consecutive patients with unstable thoracolumbar burst fractures and incomplete neurological deficits (ASIA B and C) via transpedicular decompression and instrumented fusion.[13] A canal compromise at presentation was 51.7 ± 11.2% and improved after decompression to 15.3 ± 7.8%. At an average of 14 months (range, 6–18 months) postoperatively, 14 patients improved to ASIA D and were ambulatory with an orthosis, seven patients improved to ASIA C and four patients had no improvement (ASIA B). Two patients (both ASIA B) with residual compression after the index procedure required an additional anterior decompression, with subsequent improvement to ASIA C. Vertebral height loss was 48.3 ± 7.4% preoperatively and improved to 12.7 ± 3.1% after surgery. Local kyphosis improved from 7.8 ± 2.4° preoperatively to 1.2 ± 0.8° postoperatively. There were no intraoperative complications reported. The authors contrast their minimal complications encountered using the posterior approach with those reported for the anterior approach.

Wang et al. treated 140 consecutive patients with metastatic spinal tumors necessitating circumferential decompression and instrumentation using a single-stage posterolateral transpedicular approach.[14] 96% of the patients experienced a reduction in pain and improvement in or stabilization of neurologic status. In addition, 75% of the previously nonambulatory patients (51 of 140) regained the ability to walk. At 1 month postoperatively, 90% of patients had good-to-excellent performance scores. These results demonstrate that significant palliation can be achieved through transpedicular decompression in cases of epidural tumor compression. The authors concluded that the posterolateral transpedicular approach allows for circumferential epidural tumor decompression as well as the placement of anterior and posterior column instrumentation. Furthermore, the single-stage approach avoids the morbidity associated with combined anterior-posterior approaches. The mean survival time was 7.7 months and perioperative mortality was 4.3%. No intraoperative deaths occurred in this series. The authors previously reported a 12% mortality rate in 25 patients,[15] which was reduced through medical screening and optimization.

COMPLICATIONS

Danisa et al. reported four postoperative complications in their cohort of 27 patients with unstable thoracolumbar burst fractures treated via the posterior approach. Two of their patients developed deep wound infections that were successfully treated with operative irrigation and debridement followed by 6 weeks of organism-specific antibiotics. One patient in the series developed back pain 8 months after surgery. This patient was treated with Luque instrumentation during the index procedure and was found to have protruding hardware and a pseudarthrosis. He was treated with removal of hardware, pseudarthrosis debridement and iliac crest bone grafting. Within 6 months, the patient was pain-free with radiographic fusion. One patient developed a DVT 3 weeks postoperatively and was successfully treated with pharmacologic agents.[12]

Lu et al. reported a 29% (10 of 34 patients) complication rate with no perioperative mortalities in patients undergoing transpedicular corpectomy.[9] Five patients (15%) in this group required revision surgery for a variety of reasons; one deep wound infection, two epidural hematomas, one wound dehiscence, and one kyphotic deformity distal to the instrumentation. Two patients (6%) required interventional radiologically guided drainage of epidural fluid collections.

In their series of 140 patients with epidural metastatic spine tumors, Wang et al. reported a major operative complication rate (less than 30 days postoperatively) of 14.3% (20 patients). Wound complications occurred in 16 patients (11.4%) and were not associated with postoperative radiation therapy. Only six patients in the series underwent operation within a week of radiation therapy, which may explain the lack of association. These results differ from previously reported studies.[16] Other operative complications in their series included pneumonia (2.1%), pulmonary embolism (2.1%), hematoma (0.7%), stroke (0.7%), and death (4.3%). Instrumentation failure occurred in seven patients (5%) at an average of 17 months postoperatively.

Luo et al. treated 37 patients with thoracic TB and resulting in kyphosis and spinal cord compression.[6] There were no perioperative mortalities. Perioperative complications included water-electrolyte imbalance (36 patients, 97.3%), pneumonia (six patients, 16.2%), cerebrospinal fluid leakage (two patients, 5.4%), and thrombosis (one patient, 2.7%). One patient experienced a recurrence of spinal TB and pseudarthrosis after irregular pharmacologic treatment. However, the infection resolved after abscess clearing and regular antitubercular therapy.

Mavrogenis et al. reported three complications in 25 patients with thoracolumbar burst fractures.[13] Two patients were diagnosed with superficial wound infections that resolved with local wound care and antibiotics. Deep infection occurred in one patient and required surgical debridement and antibiotics.

In a series of 59 patients, Murrey et al. reported a 16.9% complication rate.[10] Three patients experienced hardware failures; hooks cut out at the top of construct, screw loosening, and a broken rod. Two patients experienced wound infections; one superficial, one deep. One patient developed an adjacent compression fracture that required reoperation. Two patients developed pulmonary complications—respiratory failure and pulmonary edema. Other complications included transient reflex sympathetic dystrophy (now known as complex regional pain syndrome), spasticity, and hardware prominence.

CASE PRESENTATION

A 65-year-old male with a history of type 2 diabetes mellitus, hypertension, and hyperlipidemia presented to our institution with two months of worsening thoracic back pain. Subsequent workup demonstrated a hepatic mass by ultrasound as well as additional lesions in the lungs on a CT scan. The CT scan of the spine demonstrated destructive lesions involving the T8 and T9 vertebral bodies with epidural extension (Fig. 6.2).

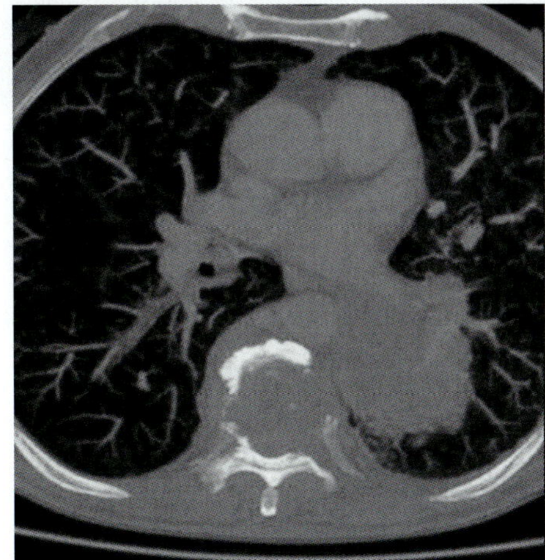
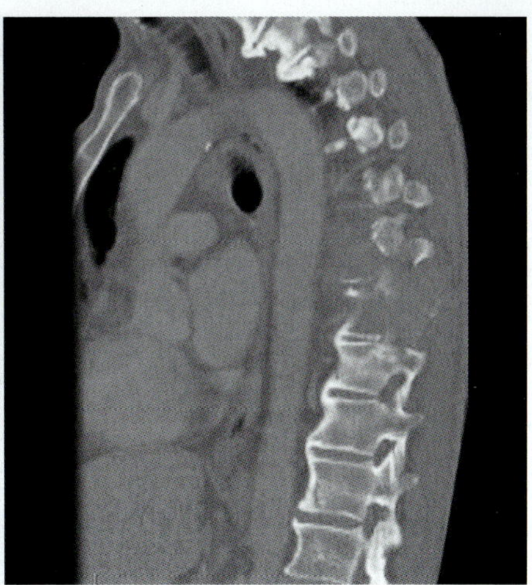

Fig. 6.2: Sagittal and axial CT scans obtained at initial presentation revealed destructive lesions involving the T8 and T9 vertebral bodies with soft extending into the spinal canal.

A physical examination demonstrated full strength in all motor groups in bilateral upper and lower extremities with intact sensation. There were no long tract signs on physical examination. An MRI revealed abnormal signal involving the T8 and T9 vertebral bodies consistent with metastatic disease and bilateral epidural extension of tumor at T8 and T9 causing spinal cord compression (Figs. 6.3 and 6.4). A biopsy of his liver mass was consistent with metastatic carcinoma. A brain MRI showed evidence of leptomeningeal metastases as well as acute lacunar infarcts. No surgical intervention was planned at this time and the patient was discharged home 1 week after initial presentation. The patient was going to continue work-up and treatment as an outpatient.

Three weeks after initial presentation, the patient returned with worsening bilateral lower extremity weakness and decreased sensation. Upon examination, the patient had decreased lower extremity sensation and reduced strength in the proximal bilateral lower extremities; 3/5 bilateral hip flexion, knee extension, 5/5 distally. The patient denied fecal/urinary incontinence and saddle anesthesia. An urgent MRI of the thoracic and lumbar spines was obtained. A repeat MRI revealed marked worsening of tumor infiltration within the T8 and T9 vertebral bodies and a progressive worsening of epidural disease and increased cord compression.

After giving consent, the patient underwent posterior spinal fusion from T5 to T12 with posterior spinal instrumentation, T7 to T10 laminectomy for removal of extradural

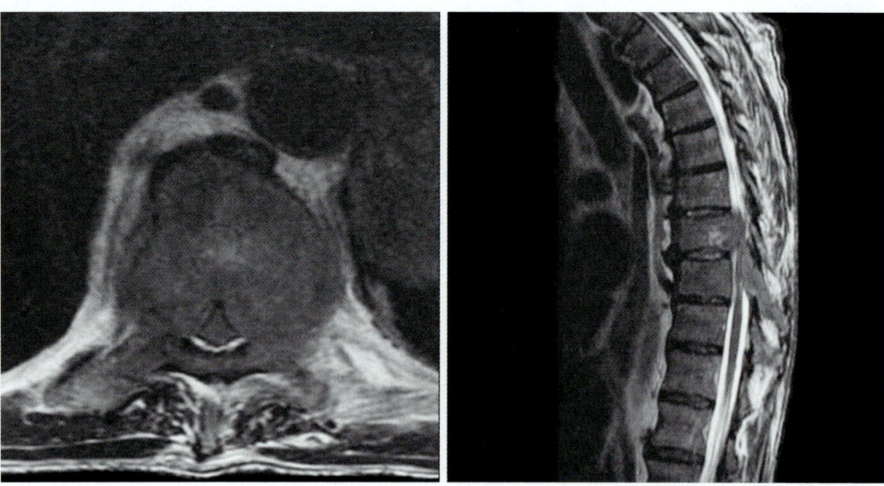

Fig. 6.3: Sagittal and axial T2-weighted MRI images obtained at initial presentation showing abnormal signal involving the T8 and T9 vertebral bodies consistent with metastatic disease and bilateral epidural extension of tumor at T8 and T9 causing spinal cord compression. The patient had normal motor and sensory examinations at this time (MRI: magnetic resonance imaging).

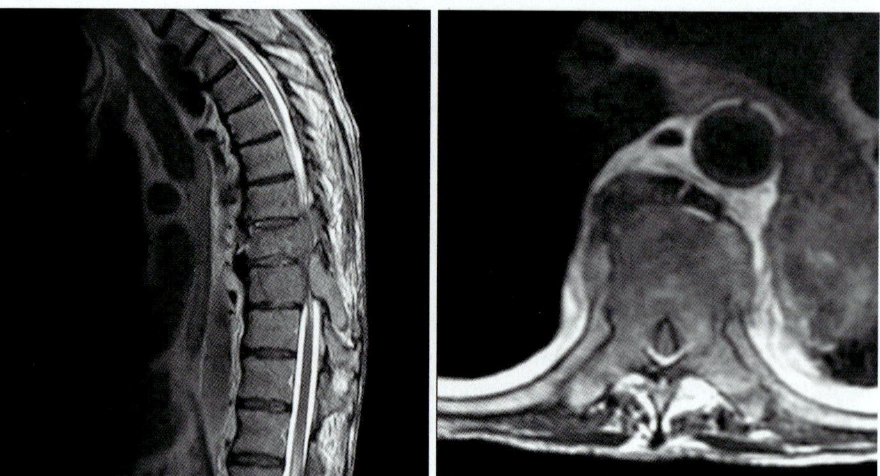

Fig. 6.4: Sagittal and axial T2-weighted MRI images obtained after neurologic decompensation showing worsening of tumor infiltration within the T8 and T9 vertebral bodies and interval worsening of epidural disease and increased cord compression (MRI: magnetic resonance imaging).

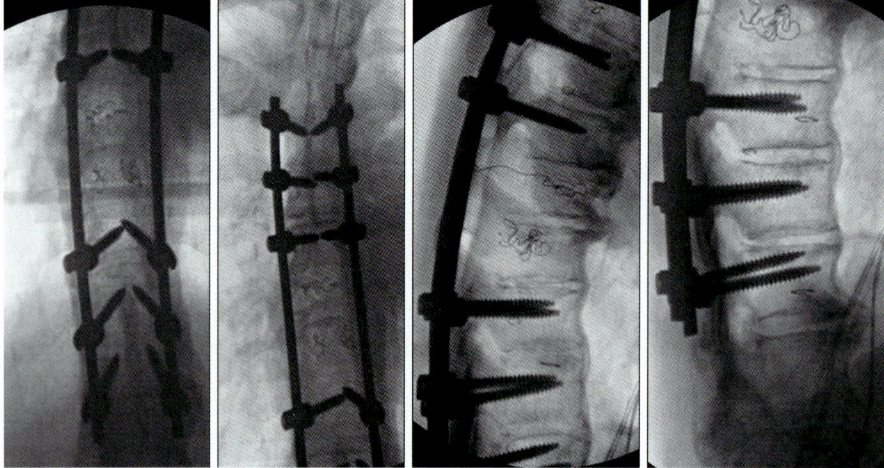

Fig. 6.5: Intraoperative radiographs. The patient underwent posterior spinal fusion from T5 to T12 with posterior spinal instrumentation, T7 to T10 laminectomy for removal of extradural mass tumor and transpedicular decompressions at T8 and T9.

mass tumor and transpedicular decompressions at T8 and T9 (Fig. 6.5). The patient required 4.5 L of crystalloid, 500 mL of albumin, two units of packed red blood cells intraoperatively and was transferred to the intensive care unit intubated. Pre- and postprocedural SSEP and MEP data was obtained in the upper extremities. There were no SSEPs in the lower extremities and motor evoked potentials were variable. The patient was extubated on postoperative day (POD) 2. The motor and sensory examinations were largely unchanged at that time. However, the patient's proximal lower extremity strength and sensation continued to improve throughout the hospital stay. Surgical pathology was consistent with metastatic squamous cell carcinoma. He was discharged to subacute rehab on POD 25 with plans for outpatient chemotherapy and external beam radiation therapy.

Case Presentation

Joshua Wynne, Joesph B Hartman, Anand Segar, Tyler Kreitz

A 69-year-old lady presented with symptoms and signs of thoracic myelopathy and difficulty ambulating. She had a known history of metastatic breast cancer. Her preoperative workup confirmed that a metastatic lesion was the cause of compression. After discussion with the patient, her husband, and her oncologist, the decision was made to proceed with decompressive surgery to ensure a sustained quality of life. The goal of surgery was not curative and no attempt was made to correct her kyphosis.

A preoperative MRI shows an anterolisthesis of T7 on T8 (Fig. 6.6). Axial images show compression at the level of the T8 vertebral body (Fig. 6.7). A preoperative CT scan confirmed the same and demonstrates bony destruction (Fig. 6.8).

The patient underwent a posterior T5-T12 fusion with a bilateral costotransversectomy, transpedicular decompression, and partial corpectomy. Both T8 nerve roots were

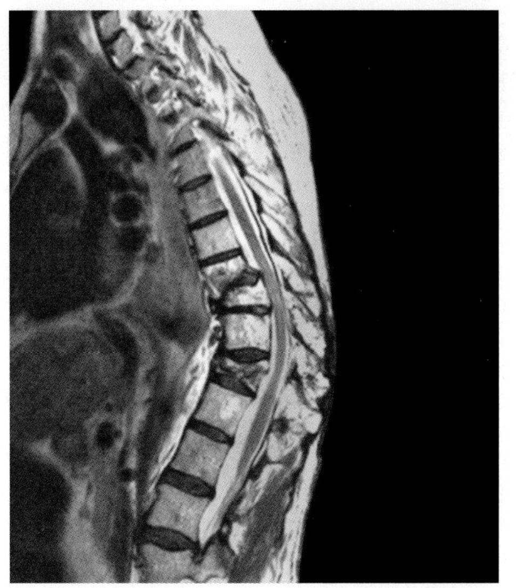

Fig. 6.6: Sagittal MRI showing cord compression at the level of T8 body (MRI: magnetic resonance imaging).

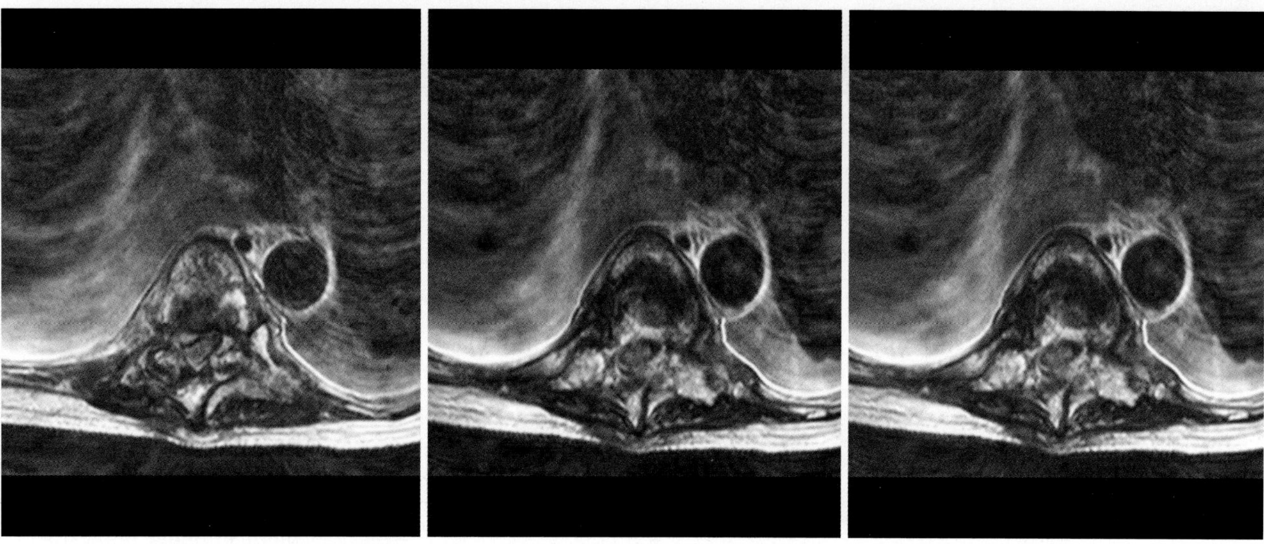

Fig. 6.7: MR axial imaging demonstrating compression behind the T7/8 disc, T8 body, and T8/9 disc.

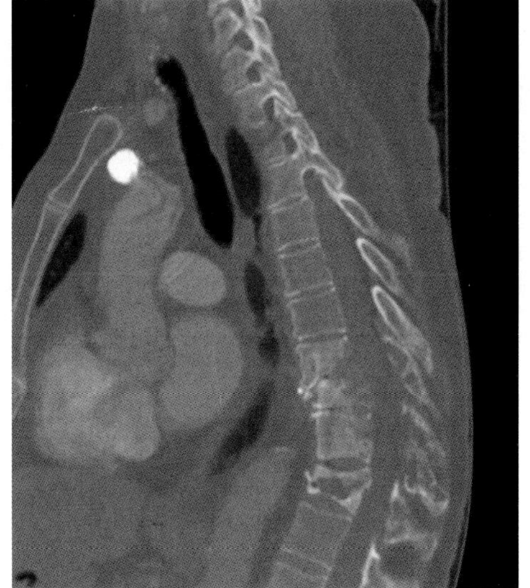

Fig. 6.8: CT sagittal image demonstrating vertebral bony destruction (CT: computed tomography).

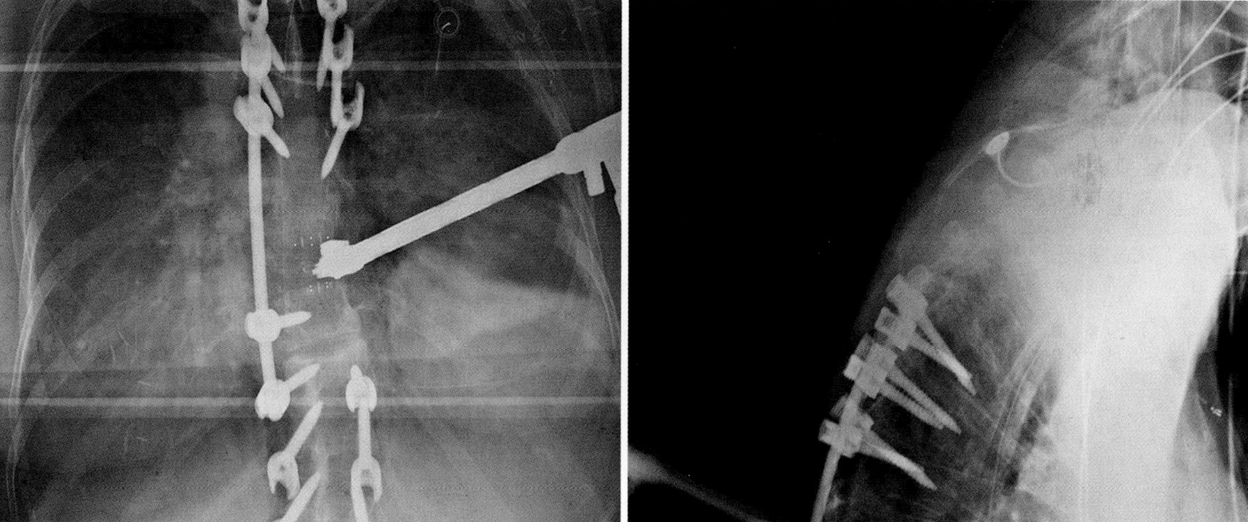

Fig. 6.9: Intraoperative anteroposterior and lateral showing cage insertion. *Courtesy:* Chris Kepler.

sacrificed to provide a surgical corridor. The vertebral body was removed from inside out burring away the cancellous bone and using a reverse angle curette to deliver the posterior vertebral wall forward into the void created within the vertebral body. An expandable polyetheretherketone (PEEK) cage was used for reconstruction and intraoperative X-rays show cage insertion. Final X-rays demonstrate the posterior instrumentation and expandable cage in situ (Figs. 6.9 and 6.10).

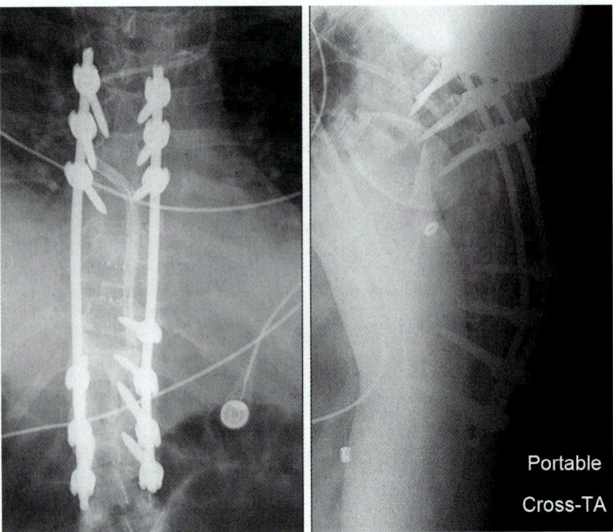

Fig. 6.10: Postoperative anteroposterior and lateral imaging.

REFERENCES

1. Fon GT, Pitt MJ, Thies AC. Thoracic kyphosis: range in normal subjects. Am J Roentgenol. 1980;134(5):979983.
2. Lauridsen KN, Carvalho AD, Andersen AH. Degree of vertebral wedging of the dorso-lumbar spine. Acta Radiologica Diagnosis. 1984;25(1):29-32.
3. Whitesides TE Jr. Traumatic kyphosis of the thoracolumbar spine. Clin Orthop Relat Res. 1977;128:78-92.
4. Chin KR. Transpedicular decompression. In: Vaccaro AR, Albert TJ (Eds). Spine Surgery: Tricks of the Trade. New York, NY: Thieme; 2009. pp. 88-9.
5. Patterson RH Jr, Arbit E. A surgical approach through the pedicle to protruded thoracic discs. J Neurosurg. 1978;48(5):768-72.
6. Luo C, Wang X, Wu P, et al. Single-stage transpedicular decompression, debridement, posterior instrumentation, and fusion for thoracic tuberculosis with kyphosis and spinal cord compression in aged individuals. Spine J. 2016;16(2):154-62.
7. Daniel S, Ikeda AM, Ramos E, et al. Surgical approaches to thoracic primary and secondary tumors. In: Kim DH (Ed). Surgical Anatomy and Techniques to the Spine. Philadelphia, PA: Elsevier Inc.; 2013. pp. 315-23.
8. Bilsky MH. Transpedicular approach for thoracic disc herniations. Neurosurgical Focus. 2000;9(4):1-4.
9. Lu DC, Lau D, Lee JG, et al. The transpedicular approach compared with the anterior approach: an analysis of 80 thoracolumbar corpectomies. J Neurosurg Spine. 2010;12(6):583-91.
10. Murrey DB, Brigham CD, Kiebzak GM, et al. Transpedicular decompression and pedicle subtraction osteotomy (eggshell procedure): a retrospective review of 59 patients. Spine (Phila Pa 1976). 2002;27(21):2338-45.
11. Wong ML, Lau HC, Kaye AH. A modified posterolateral transpedicular approach to thoracolumbar corpectomy with nerve preservation and bilateral cage reconstruction. J Clin Neurosci. 2014;21(6):988-92.
12. Danisa OA, Shaffrey CI, Jane JA, et al. Surgical approaches for the correction of unstable thoracolumbar burst fractures: a retrospective analysis of treatment outcomes. J Neurosurg. 1995;83(6):977-83.
13. Mavrogenis A, Tsibidakis H, Papagelopoulos P, et al. Posterior transpedicular decompression for thoracolumbar burst fractures. Folia Med (Plovdiv). 2010;52(4):39-47.
14. Wang JC, Boland P, Mitra N, et al. Single-stage posterolateral transpedicular approach for resection of epidural metastatic spine tumors involving the vertebral body with circumferential reconstruction: results in 140 patients. Invited submission from the Joint Section Meeting on Disorders of the Spine and Peripheral Nerves, March 2004. J Neurosurg Spine. 2004;1(3):287-98.
15. Bilsky MH, Boland P, Lis E, et al. Single-stage posterolateral transpedicle approach for spondylectomy, epidural decompression, and circumferential fusion of spinal metastases. Spine (Phila Pa 1976). 2000;25(17):2240-9.
16. Ghogawala Z, Mansfield FL, Borges LF. Spinal radiation before surgical decompression adversely affects outcomes of surgery for symptomatic metastatic spinal cord compression. Spine (Phila Pa 1976). 2001;26(7):818-24.

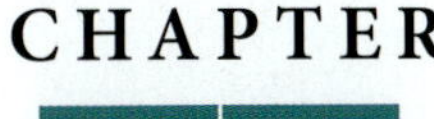

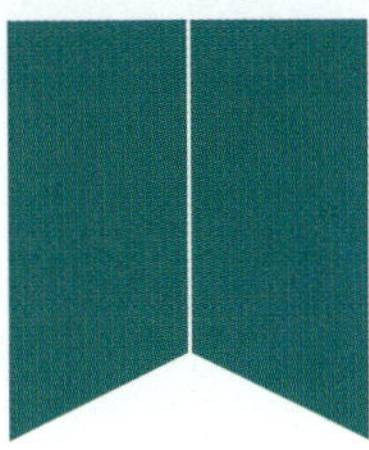

7

Multilevel Ponte Osteotomy for Thoracic Kyphosis

Arjun Sebastian, A Noelle Larson, Kyle Nappo, Scott C Wagner

ANATOMY

Thoracic spine anatomy differs in many ways compared to the cervical and lumbar spine. There are 12 thoracic vertebrae with costal facets present on the transverse processes and vertebral body. Costal facets serve as the attachment point for the rib cage. The connection of the rib cage is unique to the thoracic spine and contributes to the increased rigidity compared to the cervical and lumbar spine.[1-4]

Contrasting both the cervical and lumbar segments, the thoracic spine has a normal kyphosis, on average of 35°. Vertebral bodies in the thoracic spine increase in diameter and size as you travel cranial to caudal. However, this does not correspond to a size increase in the spinal canal diameter. Thoracic level 4, on average, has both the smallest pedicles and the shortest pedicles. This level also has the smallest canal diameter. However, more importantly is the small difference between the canal diameter and the spinal cord diameter throughout the thoracic spine. This fact is arguably the most important to take into account when evaluating pathology or surgically instrumenting the thoracic spine.[5-8]

Motion in the thoracic spine is limited secondary to facet orientation and the rigidity of the rib cage. The majority of motion is in axial rotation, and is limited in flexion and extension. Thoracic facet joints are oriented mostly in the coronal plane and allow rotation, but limited flexion and extension. This rigidity is clinically relevant in both trauma and deformity correction surgery.

In this chapter, we will be reviewing the surgical technique for multilevel Ponte osteotomies for the treatment of thoracic kyphosis.

INDICATIONS

Complex spinal deformities cause much debate on optimal management among spine surgeons. Many times, arthrodesis and instrumentation alone is not enough in order to achieve correction and restore coronal and sagittal balance. In these cases, further correction must be achieved through osteotomies. Our indication for posterior column osteotomies is a fixed kyphotic, decompensated deformity with a mobile anterior and middle column that has caused a greater than 5 mm increase in sagittal balance or loss of horizontal gaze.

A common cause of rigid thoracic kyphosis is Scheuermann's kyphosis (SK). First described in the 1920s, the condition is associated with anterior wedging of the vertebrae, end-plate irregularities, and Schmorl's nodes. Described as wedging of at least three adjacent segments of between 5° and 10°, the disease is prevalent anywhere between 0.4% and 10% of the population.[9-11] SK is typically centered with an apex in the mid-thoracic spine.[12] When SK is noted to be progressive or thoracic kyphosis is 60° or greater, generally consideration is given to an operative intervention to improve function and prevent progression of the deformity.[10,13,14]

The degree of correction must be known and the ability to hinge through the middle column must be maintained in order to have success with a posterior column osteotomy. A general rule is for every millimeter of bone that is resected, you will be able to correct 1°. On average, roughly 10 millimeters of bone is resected, resulting in roughly 10° of correction per level. However, it is imperative to note that decreases in anterior column height will decrease the degree of correction per level.

Furthermore, secondary to the rigidity of the rib cage, the degree of correction that can be expected in the thoracic spine is less than the cervical or lumbar spine. Posterior column osteotomies can be successfully performed even if coronal deformities are present.

TECHNIQUE

The Ponte osteotomy was first described to treat SK. Both Ponte and the Smith-Petersen osteotomy are posterior column wedge osteotomies that are many times used interchangeably. In fact, Ponte and colleagues[15] originally described the technique with multilevel thoracic posterior column osteotomies with posterior compression instrumentation and fusion.[15] In contrast Smith-Peterson's original technique described a posterior column osteotomy in the lumbar spine in rheumatoid patients.[16] In this chapter we refer to the Ponte osteotomy as removal of the inferior portion of the spinous process, interspinous ligament, ligamentum flavum, bilateral facet joints and inferior portion of the lamina.

Preoperative planning

As in any complex deformity case, diligent planning and an appropriately skilled and experienced surgical team is a necessity. The decisions must be made on which and how many levels will be osteotomized. The multiple levels of osteotomies allow for a gradual correction and avoid the complications of more invasive procedures. If multiple osteotomies are necessary, we recommend centering these on the apical vertebral level of the kyphotic deformity. Selection of fusion levels is critical to achieving successful deformity correction and avoiding complications related to junctional issues. The proximal extent of the fusion should include the proximal end vertebra of the kyphosis. While clearly it is imperative to extend the fusion distally to beyond the end vertebra, the ideal lower instrumented vertebra is debated.[17] Some authors advocate for inclusion of L1 versus L2 while more recent work by Cho et al.[18] has advocated for inclusion of the sagittal stable vertebra (Fig. 7.1). These authors found that stopping at this level as opposed to the first lordotic vertebra lowered the incidence of distal junctional failure.[18]

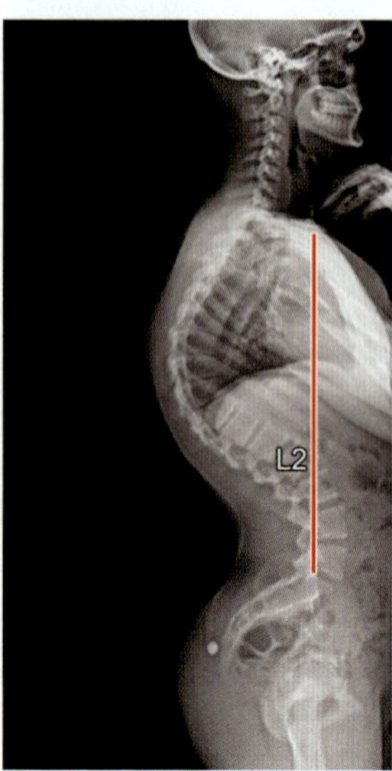

Fig. 7.1: The stable sagittal vertebra (SSV) is the most proximal vertebra touched by the posterior sacral vertical line.

Patient Positioning

Patients are placed prone on a radiolucent table and diligently positioned to reduce the risk of skin complications or brachial plexopathies. The abdomen is allowed to hang free to reduce epidural bleeding. Further, the patient is placed in cranial tongs keeping the eyes and face free, but anchoring the base of the skull in space. Positioning appropriately can reduce the risk of unnecessary complications and take advantage of any portion of the deformity that is flexible.

Intraoperative Neuromonitoring

In any deformity case, it is highly recommended to use intraoperative spinal cord monitoring. Neurologic compromise is a serious, well-known, and not so uncommon complication of complex spinal deformity correction. We routinely use somatosensory evoked potentials (SSEP), and transcranial motor evoked potentials (TC-MEP) or neurogenic mixed evoked potentials (NMEP). This allows prompt feedback if any neurologic compromise is occurring and allows the spine surgeon to appropriately react to relieve any iatrogenic spinal cord compression during reduction. Furthermore, after pedicle screw insertion stimulus triggered EMG of screws is routinely used. This form of neuromonitoring can change up to 10–15% of final screw placement. If neuromonitoring is not feasible or practical, whether secondary to resources or patient factors, wake up tests are completed to test the integrity of spinal cord tracts.

Procedure

Fluoroscopy prior to standard prepping and draping is recommended to ensure that you have adequate imaging before starting the case. Furthermore, it is imperative to use intraoperative fluoroscopy prior to completing the dissection in order to verify the planned levels for osteotomies, fusion, and instrumentation.

The standard midline posterior approach to the spine is used performing subperiosteal dissection out the ends of the transverse processes of all planned levels. At this point some surgeons choose to insert pedicle screws prior to any posterior column resection. However, many recommend placing pedicle screws after resection as this gives you visual access to the medial pedicle wall. Using this technique, one can place the pedicle screw under direct visualization to avoid breaches into the spinal canal.

Next, the inferior portion of the spinous process and the interspinous ligament is removed with a Leksell rongeur. This exposes the ligamentum flavum. Using a Kerrison rongeur, the ligamentum is taken down medially to laterally. If a coronal deformity is present, it is crucial to be particularly mindful on the concavity of the curve as this is where the spinal cord will be draped and may predispose to a dural tear. Next, the inferior articulating facet is removed with either a Kerrison rongeur or high speed burr at each level. This allows you to visualize into the canal and remove the superior articulating facet at the level of the pedicle border without violating it.

Alternatively, use of the ultrasonic bone scalpel has become more widely accepted for performing spinal osteotomies. Bartley and colleagues[19] described use of the ultrasonic bone scalpel for Ponte osteotomies. This begins with resection of the inferior articular process using two perpendicular cuts, one transverse and one longitudinal. Following this, the inferior aspect of the spinous process is resected in standard fashion using a rongeur down to the ligamentum flavum which is initially left intact. Following this the ultrasonic bone scalpel is used to osteotomize the superior articular process flush with the superior aspect of the pedicle. The ligamentum flavum is resected prior to rod insertion and deformity correction. The authors found that use of the ultrasonic bone scalpel resulted in a significant decrease in procedural blood loss of nearly 40%[19] (Figs. 7.2A to D).

Next, we prefer to place the pedicle screw on the concavity of the coronal deformity under direct visualization ensuring we avoid a medial wall breach while protecting the spinal canal. Pedicle screw placement on the convexity of the curve is done utilizing anatomic landmarks. All screws are then EMG stimulated to ensure there is not any significant medial breach.

Coronal deformity is not a contraindication to multilevel Ponte osteotomies. The coronal deformity may be corrected by differential posterior column resection on the concavity and convexity of the curve. This can be further fine-tuned at time of reduction and final instrumentation.

Once all levels have been completed and pedicle screws placed, the rods can be contoured for ideal alignment and sequential reduction can be performed to reduce the rods to the screws. Following this, sequential compression starting at the apex and working out can be performed to achieve additional correction. Aggressive cantilever reduction maneuvers should be avoided. Repeated motor evoked potentials should be performed following deformity correction to ensure no changes in neurologic status. Once satisfied with deformity correction, long intraoperative X-rays can be obtained to assess alignment. Following placement of the rods and correction, the removed bone can be morselized and laid down as fusion graft. Additionally the authors utilize morselized allograft bone for fusion as well. Alternatively, iliac crest autograft or biologics such as bone morphogenetic protein can be used for fusion.

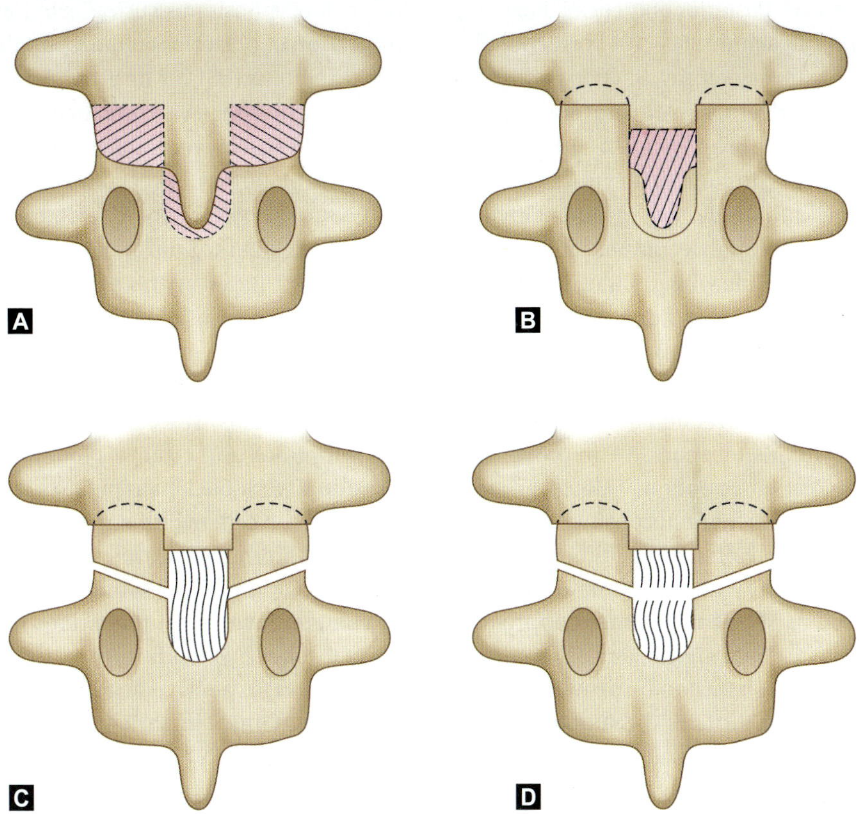

Figs. 7.2A to D: (A) Resection of the inferior articular process; (B) Resection of inferior spinous process; (C) Osteotomy of the superior articular process flush with the pedicle; and (D) Resection of the ligamentum flavum at the interspace.
Source: Bartley CE, Bastrom TP, Newton PO. Blood loss reduction during surgical correction of adolescent idiopathic scoliosis utilizing an ultrasonic bone scalpel. Spine Deform. 2014;2(4):285-90.

OUTCOMES

Although concerns regarding instrumentation failure and pseudarthrosis were described in the early literature regarding this technique, with modern pedicle screw instrumentation and more rigid fixation techniques, the posterior alone approach has become the preferred approach for most patients with SK and even more rigid thoracic kyphosis.[20-22] In a contemporary retrospective cohort of patients undergoing posterior only versus anterior-posterior treatment for SK at a high volume deformity practice, better correction and fewer complications were observed in the posterior alone group at 2 years follow-up.[20] In another retrospective cohort study of patients undergoing multilevel Ponte osteotomies and posterior fusion with pedicle screw instrumentation, Geck et al.[21] obtained good correction in all cases averaging roughly 9° of correction per level. Posterior only correction may be sufficient for kyphosis measuring up to 100° and can achieve 50–60% correction.[22] In a comparison of posterior column (Smith-Peterson osteotomy, SPO) to pedicle subtraction osteotomy (PSO), Cho et al.[23] found that the SPO achieved on average 10° of kyphosis correction per level compared to 30° for a single level PSO. The authors found that three SPOs achieved similar kyphosis correction in comparison to a single level PSO with less blood loss, lower complication rates, and similar improvement in functional outcomes. However, there was a trend toward coronal decompensation and less correction of global sagittal imbalance and C7 plumb line with multilevel SPO in comparison to PSO. Based on this evidence the authors concluded that the PSO may be recommended in cases of kyphosis where the C7 plumb line exceeds 12 cm.[23]

With regards to functional outcomes, most patients treated with osteotomy and fusion for correction of thoracic kyphosis report good results. Several studies have shown greater than 75% improvement in pain symptoms and cosmesis following surgical intervention.[24] However, some mild residual axial back pain persists into up to 65% of patients postoperatively.[25] Despite overall excellent outcomes, several studies have failed to demonstrate a clear relationship between the magnitude of deformity correction and degree of functional outcome improvement.[10,26,27] Even as surgical treatment approaches have changed over time, there does not seem to be a significant difference in functional outcomes with most patients achieving similar improvement. However, in a retrospective study by Soo et al,[27] the authors did find a trend toward poorer outcomes in patients left with a residual kyphosis of 70° or greater suggesting that there is probably a threshold of kyphosis correction that needs to be achieved for a successful functional outcome.[27]

COMPLICATIONS

The incidence of complications varies widely in the literature. In a large retrospective cohort study of over 600 patients from the Scoliosis Research Society, an overall complication rate of over 14% was determined for patients undergoing posterior fusion alone for treatment of SK.[28] The overall complication rate seems to be lower for posterior alone surgical management as opposed to anterior-posterior approaches.[20] Complications also seem to more frequent in adults compared to adolescent patients. The most common complication is surgical site infection which occurs in roughly 3–4% of cases.[28]

Certainly the most concerning potential complication with treatment of kyphosis with multilevel Ponte osteotomies is neurologic compromise. This especially true given that treatment of kyphotic deformities lengthens the spinal cord anteriorly after correction putting the anterior vascular supply at risk.[2] While most neurologic complications involve transient motor or sensory changes, spinal cord injury has been reported in 0.6% of cases with an overall neurologic complication rate of around 2%.[13,28] Preexisting stenosis may be a risk factor for neurologic injury and the authors recommend assessing and decompressing any compressive lesions prior to surgical correction. Furthermore, avoidance of overcorrection especially corrections greater than 50% is critical to preventing neurologic injury.[22,24,25] The authors also recommend multisegmental posterior compression for deformity correction as opposed to excessive cantilever reduction which can cause greater anterior distraction potentially placing the neurologic elements at risk.

In addition to careful attention to surgical techniques, the authors recommend neuromonitoring for all of these cases including both motor evoked and somatosensory potentials. Preoperative discussions and intraoperative checks with anesthesia should be undertaken to ensure adequate mean arterial pressure and oxygenation throughout the case.[21] In the event of a change in neurologic monitoring, the authors recommend a checklist approach to ensure that leads are properly positioned, mean arterial pressures are being maintained, and anesthesia is appropriate for monitoring. If changes persist, a release of the correction should be performed. In a cohort of Scheuermann's patients undergoing correction for thoracic kyphosis, Cheh et al.[29] found over a 30% incidence of loss of neuromonitoring signals following deformity correction. In all of the cases, signals improved after decreasing the correction and improving mean arterial pressure. None of the patients had neurologic deficits postoperatively.[29]

Another common and frustrating problem for surgeons treating spinal deformity is junctional kyphosis. Proximal junctional kyphosis (PJK) is defined as 10° or greater of kyphosis from the upper instrumented vertebra (UIV) to one segment cephalad. Similarly, distal junctional kyphosis (DJK) is defined as 10° of kyphosis or greater between the lower instrumented vertebra (LIV) and the next caudal segment.[13] Junctional kyphosis is a common radiographic finding. In a retrospective study of patients treated for SK, there was a 32% incidence of PJK and a 5% incidence of DJK.[13] Despite the high rate only 5% of cases were clinically significant. In another study of patients undergoing correction for SK, PJK was observed in 30% and DJK in 28% with a range of kyphosis of 10–49°.[25] Risk factors for PJK include deformity correction greater than 50% and fusing caudal to the proximal Cobb end vertebra. While some authors have advocated for the use of so called "soft landing spots" proximally either through the use of transverse process or pedicle hooks, cables or wires, or through the use of transitional rods, these techniques all have fairly mixed results regarding their efficacy in the literature. DJK rates seem to be lower when fusing to the sagittal stable vertebra. In a study by Cho et al,[18] the authors found that fusing to the sagittal stable vertebra as opposed to the first lordotic segment decreased the incidence of DJK from 71% to 4%.[18] In a similar study, Kim et al.[30] found lower revision surgery rate for DJK for patients fused to the sagittal stable vertebra as opposed to the first lordotic segment (5% vs 36%).[30]

Case Presentation

Arjun Sebastian, A Noelle Larson

Patient is a 26-year-old male with progressive axial back pain and thoracic kyphosis. This was significantly limiting his activities of daily living in addition to causing a significant cosmetic deformity. Radiographs (Figs. 7.3A and B) demonstrated a significant thoracic kyphosis of approximately 85°. Based on the patient's apex of the deformity and sagittal stable vertebrae, the levels were chosen from T2 to L3. The patient underwent posterior pedicle screw instrumentation with utilization of transverse process hooks at the proximal end of the construct to reduce junctional issues. Multilevel Ponte osteotomies were performed utilizing an ultrasonic bone scalpel from T6 to T11 (Figs. 7.4A to D). Both gentle cantilever reduction maneuvers and compression were utilized to correct the patient's deformity. Postoperative radiographs (Figs. 7.5A and B) showed good correction of the patient's kyphotic deformity.

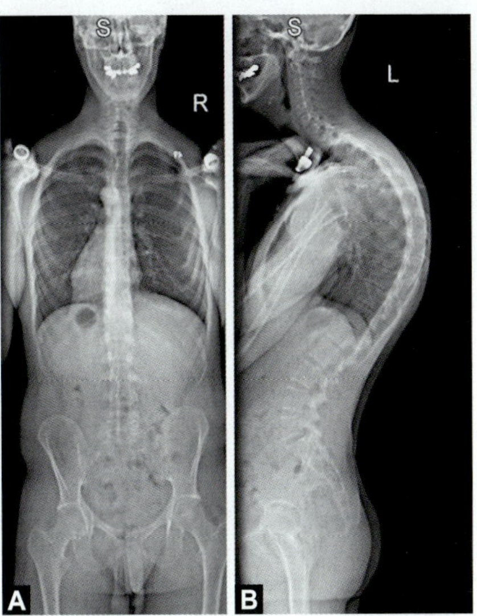

Figs. 7.3A and B: Preoperative standing AP (A) and lateral (B) radiographs demonstrating significant thoracic kyphosis.

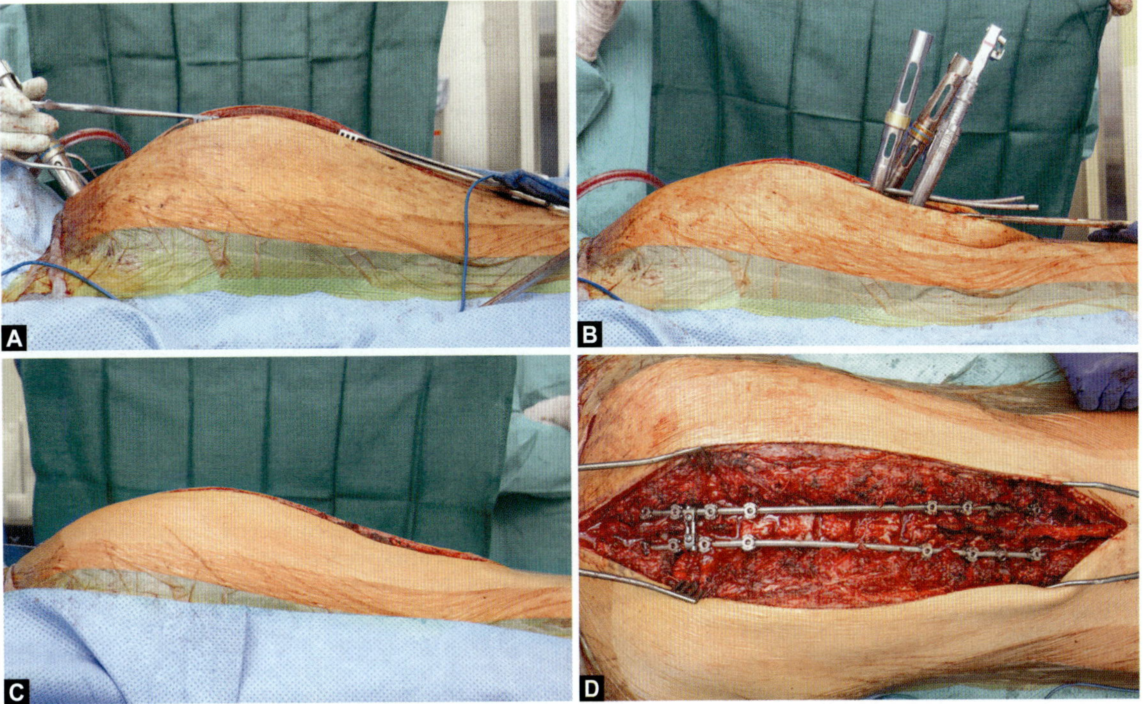

Figs. 7.4A to D: Patient's alignment prior to reduction (A). Reduction towers were utilized to help reduce the patient's deformity following the osteotomies (B). The patient's alignment was noted to be improved following reduction maneuvers (C). Posterior image demonstrating the osteotomies following correction of the deformity (D).

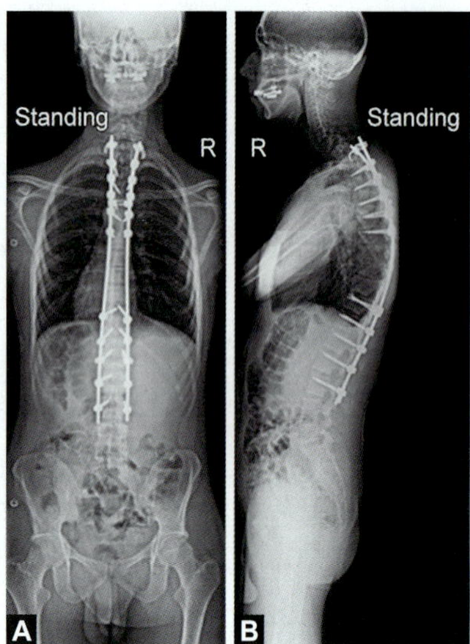

Figs. 7.5A and B: Postoperative AP (A) and lateral (B) radiographs demonstrating good correction of the patient's kyphosis.

REFERENCES

1. Magee DJ. Orthopedic Physical Assessment Enhanced edition. Amsterdam, Netherlands: Elsevier Sciences; 2006.
2. Marras WS, Simeone R. The Spine. In: Simeone R (Ed). The Spine, 6th edition. Amsterdam, Netherlands: Elsevier Health; 2011.
3. Springfield DS. Surgical Exposures in Orthopaedics: The Anatomic Approach, 4th edition. Bone. 2010.
4. Kim DH, Hen J, Vacarro AR, et al. Surgical Anatomy and Techniques to the Spine. Surg Anat Tech to Spine. 2006.
5. Berry JL, Moran JM, Berg WS, et al. A morphometric study of human lumbar and selected thoracic vertebrae. Spine (Phila. Pa. 1976). (1987).
6. Kothe R, O'Holleran JD, Liu W, et al. Internal Architecture of the Thoracic Pedicle. An Anatomic Study. Spine (Phila. Pa. 1976). 1996.
7. Panjabi MM, Takata K, Goel V, et al. Thoracic human vertebrae. quantitative three-dimensional anatomy. Spine (Phila. Pa. 1976). 1991;16(8):888-901.
8. Krag MH, Weaver DL, Beynnon BD, et al. Morphometry of the thoracic and lumbar spine related to transpedicular screw placement for surgical spinal fixation. Spine (Phila. Pa. 1976). 1988;13(1):27-32.
9. Blumenthal SL, Roach J, Herring JA. Lumbar Scheuermann's: A clinical series and classification. Spine (Phila. Pa. 1976). 1987;12(9):929-32.
10. Bradford DS, Moe JH, Montalvo FJ, et al. Scheuermann's kyphosis. Results of surgical treatment by posterior spine arthrodesis in twenty two patients. J Bone Joint Surg [Am]. 1975;57:968-72.
11. Murray PM, Weinstein SL, Spratt KE. The natural history and long-term follow-up of Scheuermann kyphosis. J Bone Joint Surg Am. 1993;75(2):236-48.
12. Ristolainen L, Kettunen JA, Kujala UM, et al. Progression of untreated mild thoracic Scheuermann's kyphosis—Radiographic and functional assessment after mean follow-up of 46 years. J Orthop Sci. 2017;22(4):652-7.
13. Lonner BS, Toombs CS, Guss M, et al. Complications in Operative Scheuermann Kyphosis: Do the Pitfalls Differ from Operative Adolescent Idiopathic Scoliosis? Spine (Phila. Pa. 1976). 2015;40(5):305-11.
14. Polly DW, Charles GTL, Beverly D, et al. What are the Indications for Spinal Fusion Surgery in Scheuermann Kyphosis? J Pediatr Orthopaed. 2017.
15. Ponte A, Orlando G, Siccardi GL. The true ponte osteotomy: by the one who developed it. Spine Deform. 2018;6(1):2-11.
16. Smith-Petersen MN, Larson CB, Aufranc OE. Osteotomy of the spine for correction of flexion deformity in rheumatoid arthritis. Clin Orthop Relat Res. 1969;66:6-9.
17. Wood KB, Melikian R, VillamilF. Adult Scheuermann kyphosis: evaluation, management, and new developments. J Am Acad Orthopaed Surg. 2012;20(2):113-21.
18. Cho KJ, Lenke LG, Bridwell KH, et al. Selection of the optimal distal fusion level in posterior instrumentation and fusion for thoracic hyperkyphosis: the sagittal stable vertebra concept. Spine (Phila. Pa. 1976). 2009;34(8):765-70.
19. Bartley CE, Bastrom TP, Newton PO. Blood loss reduction during surgical correction of adolescent idiopathic scoliosis utilizing an ultrasonic bone scalpel. Spine Deform. 2014;2(4):285-90.
20. Lee SS, Lenke LG, Kuklo TR, et al. Comparison of scheuermann kyphosis correction by posterior-only thoracic pedicle screw fixation versus combined anterior/posterior fusion. Spine. 2006;31(20):2316-21.
21. Geck MJ, Macagno A, Ponte A, et al. The ponte procedure: posterior only treatment of Scheuermann's kyphosis using segmental posterior shortening and pedicle screw instrumentation. J Spinal Disord Tech. 2007;20(8):586-93.
22. Hosman AJ, Langeloo DD, de Kleuver M, et al. Analysis of the sagittal plane after surgical management for Scheuermann's disease: a view on overcorrection and the use of an anterior release. Spine (Phila. Pa. 1976). 2002;27(2):167-75.
23. Cho KJ, Bridwell KH, Lenke LG, et al. Comparison of Smith-Petersen versus pedicle subtraction osteotomy for the correction of fixed sagittal imbalance. Spine (Phila. Pa. 1976). 2005;30(18):2030-7.
24. Lowe TG. Double L-rod instrumentation in the treatment of severe kyphosis secondary to Scheuermann's disease. Spine (Phila. Pa. 1976). 1987;12(4):336-41.
25. Lowe TG, Kasten MD. An analysis of sagittal curves and balance after Cotrel-Dubousset instrumentation for kyphosis secondary to Scheuermann's disease: a review of 32 patients. Spine (Phila. Pa. 1976). 1994;19(15):1680-5.
26. Poolman RW, Been HD, Ubags LH. Clinical outcome and radiographic results after operative treatment of Scheuermann's disease. Eur Spine J. 2002;11(6):561-9.
27. Soo CL, Noble PC, Esses SI. Scheuermann kyphosis: long-term follow-up. Spine J. 2002;2(1):49-56.
28. Coe JD, Smith JS, Berven S, et al. Complications of spinal fusion for scheuermann kyphosis: a report of the scoliosis research society morbidity and mortality committee. Spine (Phila. Pa. 1976). 2010;35(1):99-103.
29. Cheh G, Lenke LG, Padberg AM, et al. Loss of spinal cord monitoring signals in children during thoracic kyphosis correction with spinal osteotomy: why does it occur and what should you do? Spine (Phila. Pa. 1976). 2008;33(10):1093-9.
30. Kim HJ, Nemani V, Boachie-Adjei O, et al. Distal fusion level selection in Scheuermann's kyphosis: a comparison of lordotic disc segment versus the sagittal stable vertebrae. Glob Spine J. 2017;7(3):254-9.

CHAPTER

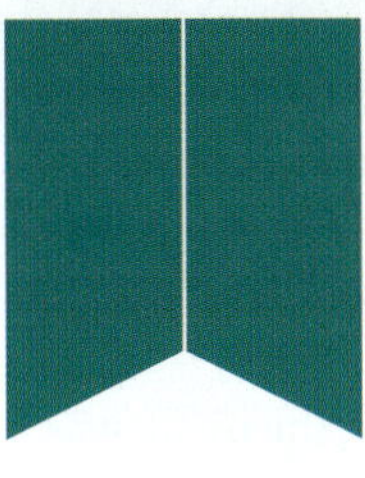

8

Vertebral Column Resection

Chris Daniels, Scott C Wagner, Larry Lenke

ANATOMY

Vertebral column resection (VCR), as defined by Lenke et al.[1], is a three-column circumferential vertebral osteotomy creating a segmental defect with sufficient instability to require provisional instrumentation. It completely separates the spinal column into two limbs, and is the most powerful corrective technique reserved only for severe spinal deformity. Resection is performed at the apex of the deformity, and is indicated for severe, rigid scoliotic and kyphotic spinal deformities. In this setting, a thorough understanding of the anatomy of the rotated vertebral segments is critical, and the surgeon must appreciate the morphologic and iatrogenic changes of the posterior elements, as well as the course of the spinal cord and nerve roots.

The spinous process, lamina, transverse processes, and facet joints of the vertebra in the fusion range are subperiosteally exposed by a standard midline incision during the surgical procedure. In the thoracic spine, the rib heads may also be resected. In the thoracic spine, the aorta is immediately anterior to the vertebral column distal to T5. However, this normal relationship may be distorted in severe spinal deformity. The segmental arteries to the vertebral bodies must be identified and ligated about the spinal segment to be resected.

INDICATIONS

Indications for a VCR can be divided into five diagnostic categories—(1) kyphoscoliosis, (2) severe scoliosis, (3) congenital deformity, (4) global kyphosis, and (5) angular kyphosis. The findings of a retrospective cohort of patients who underwent posterior-only VCR (pVCR)[1] suggest that the procedure may be indicated in patients with kyphoscoliosis for a preoperative maximum sagittal Cobb angle greater than 40°. Global kyphosis greater than 65° and angular kyphosis greater than 40, severe scoliosis with a preoperative coronal Cobb angle more than 50°, or congenital deformity can also be treated with a posterior VCR. While the Cobb method is a useful comparison metric, the radiographical measures in these cases often under-represent the deformity and the benefit of the VCR procedure for these patients.

The location and the number of vertebrae removed are determined by the type of the deformity and the desired correction to restore the trunk balance. In kyphoscoliosis, the fusion level includes one level above the upper end vertebra of index curve to one level caudal to the lower end vertebra of the index curve. For patients with kyphosis, consider fusion of three vertebrae above the resection to two vertebrae below the resection.

Preoperative Planning

A thorough history and physical examination are essential. Some patients with severe deformities can present with neurologic dysfunction. In the pediatric population, genetic, neurologic, hematologic, pulmonary, and endocrine consultations may be indicated based on previous diagnoses and current health problems. Many of these patients have significant respiratory compromise secondary to their deformities, and it is common to have poor function and diminished pulmonary reserve. Thus, all deformity patients should undergo pulmonary consultation and training prior to surgery. Of note, patients with pulmonary limitations are more able to tolerate a modern surgery using a posterior-only approach compared to an open anterior approach or thoracotomy. A complete laboratory evaluation should be performed, including a platelet function panel, complete blood count, nutritional values, and chemistry panel. Blood products must be available for use intraoperatively. By establishing baseline parameters for each patient's general medical health, adjustments and improvements can be made to preoperative preparation on an individualized basis.

Standard initial workup for patients suffering from severe spinal deformity involves upright coronal and sagittal plane radiographs. However, given the complex three-dimensional (3-D) deformities of these patients, vertebral landmarks are often poorly visualized and more advanced imaging is mandatory. Obtaining a 3-D computed tomography (CT) scan allows for delineation of the deformity and detailed examination of the bony anatomy, including any deficiencies in the posterior column, which may predispose the patient to dural laceration during the exposure. In revision cases and those with congenitally altered vertebral structures, obtaining a life-sized model of the entire spinal column can be extremely beneficial to study preoperatively and to have available intraoperatively using a sterile plastic cover. The entire neural axis from the craniocervical junction to the sacrum should undergo magnetic resonance imaging (MRI), as it is not uncommon for neuroanatomic abnormalities (including a tethered spinal cord or Chiari malformations) to be associated with bony deformities of the spinal column. If present, these anomalies should prompt evaluation by neurological surgery prior to the proposed deformity correction surgery.

Preoperative optimization of all medical comorbidities and other parameters is strongly encouraged. Presurgical hospitalization also provides opportunities for the patient to receive appropriate nutritional support, exercise, and physical therapy as well as daily respiratory therapy. Structured ambulation programs can maximize pulmonary and cardiac capacity. Patients with severe nutritional deficiencies can receive enteral or parenteral nutrition, and preliminary gastrostomy tubes or central venous access can be placed if necessary. For pediatric patients, halo traction prior to surgery can allow for gradual safe elongation of the spinal column and neural axis. Intubation is often very difficult in patients with cervicothoracic deformities, and thorough preoperative evaluation by the anesthesia team is mandatory as a fiber-optic intubation may be required.

SURGICAL TECHNIQUE

The surgical techniques employed during a posterior VCR are technically demanding, and is typically performed only by experienced surgical teams.[2,3] The operating surgeon should have a baseline comfort level with posterior three-column pedicle subtraction, posterior hemivertebra resection, costotransversectomies, and comfort with handling the dural sac—including removing adhesions, fibrous tissue, or epidural fat over multiple levels of the dura. Performing this type of complicated spinal deformity surgery carries significant risk to the patient, and the learning curve for the surgeon is steep.

Vertebral column resection was first illustrated by MacLennan for the treatment of severe scoliosis in 1922.[4] VCR was performed as described by Bradford through a combined anterior and posterior approach in 1987,[5] and became a viable option for the surgical management of severe deformities with the development of segmental instrumentation. Resection of the vertebral body and discs were performed through a formal anterior approach, with removal of the posterior elements and posterior instrumentation and fusion from the posterior approach.[6]

To mitigate complications of anterior and posterior VCR, the pVCR was introduced in 2002.[7] pVCR allows the procedure to complete in one stage, thus reducing overall operative time and blood loss, and also providing the greatest amount of surgical correction when compared to all other spinal osteotomy techniques.[6] The pVCR is a significantly more powerful corrective technique compared to pedicle subtraction osteotomy (PSO) as the surgeon gains complete control of the proximal and distal segments of the deformity by essentially disarticulating the spinal column.[8]

Spinal Cord Monitoring

Sensory and motor tract monitoring should be provided throughout the duration of these neurologically high-risk surgeries, and the spinal cord monitoring team must be attentive during all stages of the procedure. Intraoperatively, somatosensory evoked potentials (SSEP), and either transcranial motor evoked potentials (TC-MEP) or neurogenic mixed evoked potentials (NMEP) are used. Spinal motor conduction can quickly and accurately be evaluated by TC-MEP.[9] Use of upper extremity SSEPs can prevent brachial plexopathies. Electromyography (EMG) used in a spontaneous elicited fashion (primarily for procedures involving the lumbar spine) also provides helpful information to monitor the lumbar nerve roots. Normally, we also use stimulus triggered EMGs of pedicle screws in the thoracic spine from T6 to T12 and the entire lumbar spine to evaluate for any violation of the pedicle wall into the canal.

Anesthesia Considerations

Many of these patients are at high risk for neurologic injury secondary to chronic myelopathy or possible ligation of segmental vessels after previous surgery, so optimizing spinal cord perfusion intraoperatively is imperative. A normotensive blood pressure with mean arterial pressure (MAP) of approximately 70–80 mm Hg should be maintained. When treating severe angular kyphosis, a minimum MAP of 80 mm Hg is ideal throughout the entire procedure, and higher during the most critical portions of the VCR. During actual closure of the resected area, a mean pressure of more than 80 mm Hg is preferred for all patients. It is also extremely important that the anesthesia team remain acutely aware of the likelihood for significant blood loss during the procedure, and various antifibrinolytics are advised to aid in decreasing blood loss. Use of tranexamic acid (TXA), at a 100 mg/kg loading dose and 10 mg/kg maintenance dose, can decrease blood loss 25–50% intraoperatively.[10]

Surgical Procedure

For the pVCR, the patient is placed in the prone position on a radiolucent operating table after induction of general anesthesia. Depending on the size of the patient and the nature of the deformity, a halo or Gardner-Wells tongs with traction may be placed in the operating room. Doing so allows the skull to be anchored while the face and eyes remain free, but excessive traction should be avoided in patients with severe kyphotic deformities. Keeping the abdomen free and the arms abducted and externally rotated and well-padded minimizes the risk of skin injuries, brachial plexopathies, and peripheral neuropathies. Proper positioning of patients with severe deformities is particularly important, albeit time consuming.

After identifying the vertebral levels to be addressed, the spinous process, lamina, transverse processes, and facet joints of the vertebra in the fusion range are subperiosteally exposed by a midline incision. Some cases require exposure of the sacrum and/or ilium. At the apex of the thoracic deformity, it is not uncommon to perform convex medial rib thoracoplasties to gain adequate exposure of the convex transverse processes.

Following exposure, multilevel posterior column osteotomies (Ponté- or Smith-Petersen-type) are performed around the apex of the deformity. Performing multilevel posterior column osteotomies increases the flexibility of the periapical region, thereby allowing for more harmonious correction once the resection is complete. Every level is individually notched and 3–4 mm of the inferior facet is removed. The ligamentum flavum is excised and the proximal portion of the superior articular facet is removed above the pedicle within the foramen over the levels to be osteotomized. This maneuver also decreases the risk posed by periapical pedicle screw placement; since these vertebrae are often severely deformed, exposing the spinal canal following the osteotomy allows palpation of the medial border of the pedicle and prevents potentially catastrophic placement of the concave screws in the canal. Pedicle screws are placed prior to performing the osteotomies only if the patient has severe angular kyphosis. Routinely, temporary stabilizing rods are placed prior to any posterior column destabilization because there is a risk of ventral migration of the spinal column and impingement on the spinal cord.

The efficient and safe placement of pedicle screws is a critical component and typically proceeds from distal to proximal. Consider segmental fixation with placement of many periapical screws to provide stability near the planned resection site, utilizing free-hand technique and a blunt gearshift to place screws. In patients with a prior fusion mass at the apex of their deformity, do not attempt apical concave screw placement without having prior access of the spinal canal and medial pedicle border through a laminectomy or laminotomy at the apex. Placement of convex thoracic periapical screws in fusion masses is typically safe because the spinal cord is usually distant from the convex pedicle site. Depending on surgeon preference and experience level, consider fluoroscopic and image guidance techniques for safe and efficacious screw placement. Multiaxial screws or multiaxial reduction screws (MARS) are recommended at the immediately adjacent levels of the resection site, as these screws allow for efficient placement of temporary rods around the apex and the ends of kyphotic deformities, and can aid in reducing any subluxations that may occur. After placement of all screws, intraoperative anteroposterior and lateral radiographs are obtained to confirm and document accurate screw placement. EMG is performed for all screws placed from T6 to S1. In ambulatory patients fused to the sacrum and ilium, adjunctive transforaminal lumbar interbody fusion (TLIF) confers anterior structural support and supports fusion of the lumbosacral disc.

At the level of planned thoracic vertebra resection, bilateral costotransversectomies should be performed. To avoid inadvertent canal intrusion, remove 5 cm of the associated medial rib prior to the laminectomy using circumferential, subperiosteal dissection of the rib. Maintain these ribs whole and not morselized, as they will be used to cover the laminectomy defect at the end of the procedure and provided structural bone graft to the area. Next, a complete laminectomy from the inferior pole of the pedicles above the resection to the superior pole of the pedicles below the resection should be performed. In a characteristic adolescent or adult patient undergoing a single-level resection, this action will result in approximately a 5 cm laminectomy defect. Identify the entire dural sac through this exposure and free any fibrous tissue, adhesions, or epidural fat. At this point, the thoracic nerve root on the convex side of the apical vertebra to be resected is typically ligated. Although not absolutely necessary, doing so makes the remainder of the vertebral resection easier. Temporarily clamp the nerve root and perform continuous spinal cord monitoring for 5–10 min to verify that there is no diminution in spinal cord blood supply. If monitoring remains stable during clamping of the nerve root, then double tie the root as medial to the dural sac as possible and transect it. Ligation of multiple thoracic roots unilaterally does not cause neurologic compromise, or sensory deficit to the chest wall—provided less than four roots are ligated. Preserve the concave roots if possible, and always maintain the roots in the lumbar spine (Figs. 8.1A to F).

A temporary stabilizing rod is attached to, at a minimum, two pedicle screws both above and below the resection area. Classically, a unilateral rod is used; however, in severe angular kyphotic or kyphoscoliotic deformities, bilateral rods are recommended to prevent subluxation of the spinal column. The pedicles to be resected are encircled, and the vertebral body resection begins by gaining access to its cancellous bone through a lateral pedicle-body entrance. Curette the cancellous bone of the vertebral body, and save all removed bone for graft. For a patient with pure scoliosis or kyphoscoliosis, the majority of the vertebral body will be removed from the convexity of the deformity. Resecting the apical concave pedicle can be quite challenging. The pedicle encountered during this step tends to be extremely cortical, and often the entire dural sac rests on the medial concave pedicle. However, the pedicle on the concavity may not even have an associated ventral vertebral body, as it is often rotated laterally and dorsally on the convexity of the deformity. Utilize a

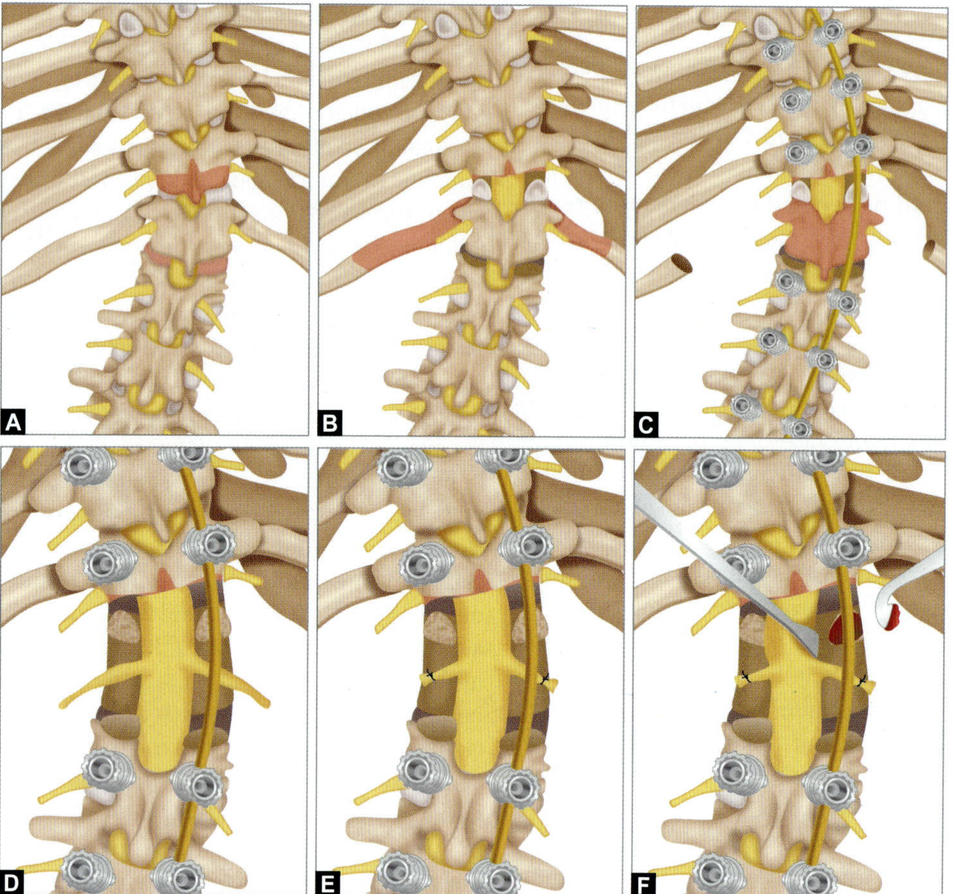

Figs. 8.1A to F: (A) Inferior facetectomies are performed to gain flexibility and assist with pedicle screw placement; (B) Costotransversectomy is performed bilaterally prior to laminectomy resecting approximately the medial 5 cm of the rib; (C) Laminectomy is performed with resection of the superior articular facet above and below to expose the spinal cord and nerve root exiting caudal to the targeted pedicle; (D) Following pedicle screw placement a temporary rod is inserted for stabilization; (E) The nerve roots are then ligated bilaterally to improve exposure; (F) The pedicles should be resected and the vertebral body decancellated with use of curettes and a high-speed burr.
Source: https://www2.aofoundation.org/wps/portal/surgery?showPage=diagnosis&bone=Spine&segment=Overview

small, high-speed burr to remove the cortical bone along the concavity of the deformity while protecting the adjacent dural sac and spinal cord. By performing the concave resection of the pedicle prior to the convexity, bleeding into the dependent concave region is minimized. Doing so also allows the concave dural sac to drift medially, thereby reducing tension on the cord prior to completion of the vertebrectomy. Following subperiosteal exposure of the lateral portion of the vertebral body and placement of a malleable or customized "spoon" retractors to protect the adjacent vascular structures and viscera, remove the entire body except for the anterior shell. Maintaining a thin rim of bone on the anterior longitudinal ligament (ALL), in theory, improves fusion. However, the anterior bone must be thinned, if very dense, to allow closure of the resection area.

Discectomies above and below the corpectomy site are now performed. The endplates of the superior and inferior adjacent vertebral bodies must be kept intact, as placement of a structural intracorporeal cage may be required. Epidural hemostasis can be achieved through the judicious use of bipolar cauterization, topical hemostatic agents, and cottonoids. Removal of the posterior vertebral body wall or floor of the spinal canal may then proceed. The dural sac must be exposed circumferentially and separated from the epidural venous complex, as well as from the posterior longitudinal ligament (PLL). The posterior vertebral wall may be removed in its entirety with reverse-angled curettes, Kerrison rongeurs, Woodson elevators, or specialized posterior wall impactors. The ventral spinal cord must be completely free of any bony prominences to avoid impingement during closure of the osteotomy. Osteophytosis of the adjacent disc levels may cause ventral compression, and any bony prominences at these levels must be resected carefully.

Once the vertebral resection is complete, closure of the resected area begins with compression forces applied on the convexity, with initial shortening of the spinal. In cases with good bone stock, this technique is performed with individual pedicle screws. Alternatively, a construct-to-construct closure mechanism may utilize domino connectors at the apex of the resected area. This method distributes the forces of correction over several vertebral levels, and functions in a stepwise fashion by closing the osteotomy from a construct rod above to a construct rod below. It is imperative to compress deliberately, and to monitor the dural sac as vertebral subluxation or dural impingement can occur during this step of the operation. If the patient has a kyphotic deformity, place an anterior structural cage to prevent over-shortening of the deformity and to act as a fulcrum to aid further correction. The placement of an intervertebral cage provides shear force stabilization by the interdigitation of the cage into the endplates facilitating anterior fusion. Once the closure has been completed and appropriate correction maneuvers performed, a permanent contralateral rod is placed. The temporary closing rod is removed and a permanent rod is placed on the ipsilateral side. Appropriate compression and distraction forces, in situ contouring, and other correction techniques may be performed. A careful and repetitive palpation of the dural sac circumferentially is performed at every iterative step of the correction to confirm that it is not undergoing undo tension, impingement, or buckling (Figs. 8.2A to F).

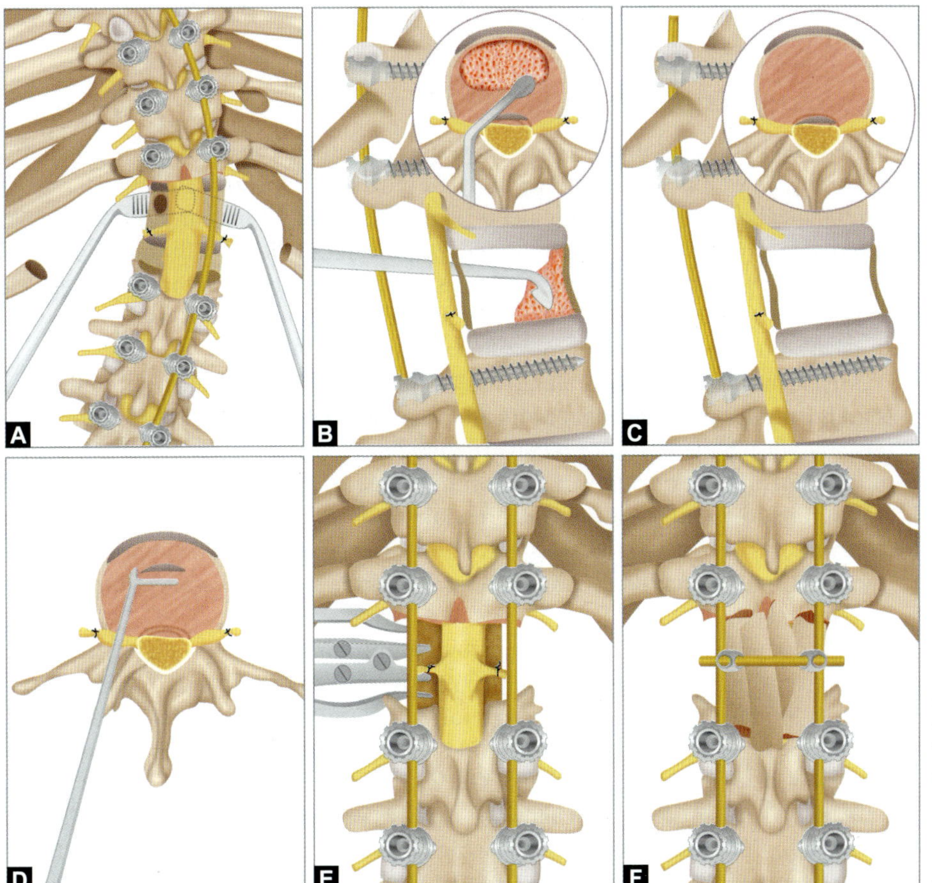

Figs. 8.2A to F: (A) Following pedicular resection and decancellation of the posterior body, lateral subperiosteal dissection is performed and spoon-tye retractors are placed to protect the anterior structures; (B) Decancellation is continued in the body using a combination of curettes and rongeurs lateral and ventral to the cord; (C) Decancellation is continued until the anterior vertebral body margin is reached. (D) The final step in the osteotomy requires tamping forward of the remaining posterior cortex; (E) Following this, a vertebral cage, or structural bone graft may be placed into the void to reconstruct the anterior and middle columns; (F) The resected ribs from the costotransversectomy may be used to cover the laminectomy defect.
Source: https://www2.aofoundation.org/wps/portal/surgery?showPage=diagnosis&bone=Spine&segment=Overview

Adequate alignment is confirmed by intraoperative radiographs. Decortication and bone grafting follow, using local graft obtained from the resection procedure. The laminectomy defect is covered with the previously harvested ribs from the costotransversectomy. Preferentially, the ribs are cut longitudinally, and the cancellous surface is placed along the entire laminectomy defect. This structural grafting of the laminectomy protects the dura and provides a posterior onlay fusion. The rib graft is held in place with sutures or a crosslink. Lastly, confirm the absence of any dural impingement, document final implant security, and confirm intact spinal cord monitoring. The incision should be closed over suction drains, and an intraoperative wake-up test may be performed to ensure maintenance of neurologic status prior to extubation. Before exiting the operating room, final radiographs are obtained to verify radiographic deformity correction.

OUTCOMES

A major curve correction utilizing the pVCR in patients has been reported to range from 51 to 60%, or 62 and 72% in the coronal and sagittal planes, respectively, depending on the patient population and type of deformity.[18,19] Other reported rates of correction include 54% for global kyphosis, 56% for kyphoscoliosis, 63% for angular kyphosis, and 69% for scoliosis.[2,11,12] When compared to published correction values of 30º to 40º for pedicle subtraction osteotomies or other closing wedge osteotomies,[13] pVCR is a significantly more powerful technique for deformity correction.

While pVCR allows for reduction in operative time and estimated blood loss (EBL) versus a combined VCR approach, the procedure is still associated with substantial surgical time and potential morbidity. An average operative time has been reported from 8 hours[12] to 10 hours, with ranges approaching 24 hours.[3] The average EBL ranges from 250 mL to 3,100 mL,[3] with mean percent of blood loss in one series averaging 76%.[14] Intraoperative blood loss as high as 24 L, have also been reported.[15,16] However, Auerbach et al.[17] found that when compared directly to PSO, pVCR yielded a lower average intraoperative blood loss. Neuromuscular disease in pediatric patients is a risk factor for intraoperative loss of greater than 50% of the circulating blood volume.[14] Hospital stay averages 14 days in pediatric neuromuscular patients (ranging up to 40 days), with 6 days spent in the intensive care unit (ICU),[14] on average.

Pulmonary function testing (PFT) improves after deformity correction,[15] though improvements in adults may be diminished when compared to pediatric patients. When compared to anterior surgery with thoracotomy, the immediate deterioration in pulmonary function postoperatively is lowered in patients undergoing posterior-only procedures. This finding suggests that, in pediatric patients with severe restrictive pulmonary disease, posterior-only procedures are preferred.[18] Both mean forced vital capacity (FVC) and forced expiratory volume in 1 s (FEV1) have shown improvement after pVCR in pediatric patients.[19] The degree of improvement may correlate with younger age at the time of surgery, diagnosis of angular kyphosis, no previous spine surgery, and the use of preoperative halo traction.[19]

Patients undergoing the surgery have shown significant improvements noted in reported patient self-image, pain, and functional scores when compared to their preoperative Scoliosis Research Society (SRS) scores.[17] Patient satisfaction is observed despite the occurrence of complications, and improvements in patient-reported outcomes and radiographic alignment are maintained at 5-year follow-up.[20]

COMPLICATIONS

The reported overall complication rate has ranged widely, from 7.84[11] to 59%.[1,2,14,17,21] Associated risk factors for perioperative complications have been shown to include patient age greater than 60 years, associated medical comorbidities, and obesity.[22] Major and minor complications can be subdivided into neurologic and non-neurologic complications. The overall revision rate after VCR is as high as 22.2%. Patients must be counseled preoperatively that these risks are significant, and the benefits of surgery must be carefully weighed.

Neurologic Complications

There is high inherent neurologic risk, partially related to the severity of the spinal deformity, as well as the instability induced during correction.[23] The overall rate of neurological deficit has recently been reported at 5.6%,[17] compared to previously reported rates of dysfunction in 17, 22, and 29% in other studies.[2,8,24] The most common intraoperative complication for pVCR is the loss of spinal cord monitoring data, which occurs in as many as 75% of pVCR cases,[25] and approximately 10–15% of cases require surgical adjustment after a neuromonitoring change.[1,17]

Given the significant neurologic risk inherent in pVCR, spinal cord monitoring is mandatory during deformity reduction maneuvers. The spine is rendered highly unstable during the posterior reconstruction, and it is not uncommon for patients to lose NMEP data during this portion of the case, often secondary to vertebral subluxation, dural buckling, or compression of the cord by residual tissue after the deformity has been corrected.[3,6] NMEP data loss can be addressed via improvement in the MAP, thorough ventral decompression, and/or through restoration of appropriate anterior height.

In those patients with previously treated intraspinal anomalies, such as tethered cord or intraspinal tumors—or even in patients with a coexistent conditions such as Charcot-Marie-Tooth disease—intraoperative monitoring may be unobtainable, and spinal cord or nerve root dysfunction can be diagnosed by a wake-up test during the procedure.[1]

Patients with severe kyphoscoliosis or kyphosis with prior anterior fusion surgery in the context of thoracic myelopathy are at higher risk for major neurologic compromise postoperatively.[17] Similarly, preoperative neurologic deficit is a significant risk factor for neurologic sequelae in the postoperative period, and must be carefully considered and discussed with each individual patient.[21,25] Risk factors for neurological complications include age ≥ 18, pulmonary dysfunction, and blood loss more than 50% of circulating volume.[26]

Suk and colleagues[7] reported complete spinal cord injuries in two patients, although their series included patients being monitored with SSEPs alone. Kim et al.[21] reported a 3.3% rate of permanent neurologic deficit, and an 11.2% rate of dural tear with pVCR. Another series reported gait deterioration in two of 11 patients with chronic gait disturbances postoperatively.[8] Wang et al.[25] published a series of 77 pVCR procedures, noting that 37 (48%) cases showed obvious monitoring degenerations, and 21 (27%) cases had significant monitoring loss. Overall, three (4%) patients had a new spinal deficit at 1-year follow-up. While the risk of catastrophic neurologic injury remains very high with this procedure, it is likely—though difficult to prove directly—that spinal cord monitoring and intraoperative protocols have dramatically reduced the incidence of these complications.[1,12]

Non-neurologic Complications

Postoperative pulmonary complications are common, likely related to the thoracic insufficiency and anatomic deformities present in these patients.[1] Pneumothorax has been reported, and chest tubes may be placed in a prophylactic manner if the risk of pneumothorax is high. Xie et al.[15] reported that in their series of 28 patients with severe (greater than 100° thoracic or thoracolumbar Cobb angle) thoracic or thoracolumbar deformities, three patients sustained acute pulmonary edema intraoperatively, three patients developed postoperative pneumonia, and eight patients had chest tubes placed.

Posterior wound infection rates have been reported at 4%,[1] though wound infections deep to the fascia are uncommon.[7,24,27] However, a study reported by Papadopoulos et al.[8] reported a surgical debridement rate of 8.9% after a major posterior spinal deformity surgery.

In the series by Wang et al.[28], 14% of cases were complicated by rod breakage at the level of osteotomy at a mean of 6.8 months (range 5–12 months) after surgery. They noted that risk factors included body mass index (BMI) more than 27 kg/m^2, achondroplasia, and anterior column defects greater than 20 mm.

CASE PRESENTATION

The patient is a 16-year-old female with neurofibromatosis, 4 years status post combined anterior and posterior spinal fusion for neuromuscular scoliosis, with progressive kyphoscoliosis and mild myelopathy after implant removal for proximal prominence. An upright anteroposterior (Fig. 8.3A) and lateral (Fig. 8.3B) radiographs demonstrated a 61° main thoracic and 35° lumbar scoliosis curves, with 180° thoracic kyphosis. A preoperative 3-D CT reconstructions (Figs. 8.4A to D) showed severe vertebral wedging and a complex sagittal deformity. A T2-weighted MRI demonstrated dural ectasia and spinal cord impingement (Figs. 8.5A to C), consistent with the patient's myelopathic symptoms. Preoperative PFT revealed an FVC of 23.4% predicted, and a FEV1 of 25.3% predicted, indicative of severe restrictive pulmonary disease. The patient was placed in hanging traction with 20 pounds for over 3 months, with improvements in her radiographic alignment (Figs. 8.6A and B) and a 10% improvement in pulmonary function. She also had a Broviac catheter placed for total parenteral nutrition (TPN) to optimize her nutritional status prior to the surgery. Clinical photos (Figs. 8.7A to C) show improvement in the curve over the course of hanging traction.

The procedure was performed in a staged fashion. During stage 1, a wide posterior exposure was performed making every effort to minimize blood loss (Fig. 8.8). Pedicle screws were placed free-hand, and a 3-D resin model of the patient's spine was utilized as a guide throughout this aspect of the procedure (Fig. 8.9). A temporary concave rod was placed for stabilization (Fig. 8.10). Stage 2 began with apical spinal cord exposure, decompression, and vertebral body resection (Figs. 8.11A to D). After cantilever correction of the deformity via posterior compression and anterior distraction (Fig. 8.12), the laminectomy defect from the VCR is covered with structural rib graft (Fig. 8.13). Final postoperative radiographs and clinical images are shown in Figures 8.14A to D. The patient's neurologic function recovered fully 4 weeks postoperatively.

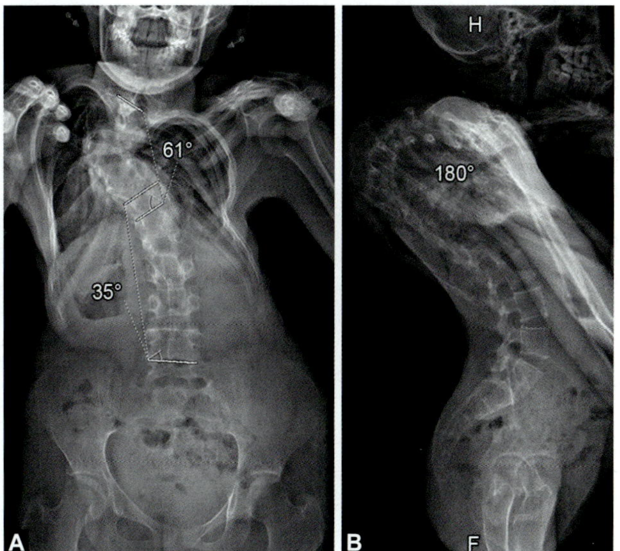

Figs. 8.3A and B: The patient is a 16-year-old female with neurofibromatosis; 4 years status post-combined anterior and posterior spinal fusion for neuromuscular scoliosis, with progressive kyphoscoliosis and mild myelopathy after implant removal for proximal prominence. Upright anteroposterior (A) and lateral (B) radiographs demonstrated a 61° main thoracic and 35° lumbar scoliosis curves, with a 180° thoracic kyphosis.

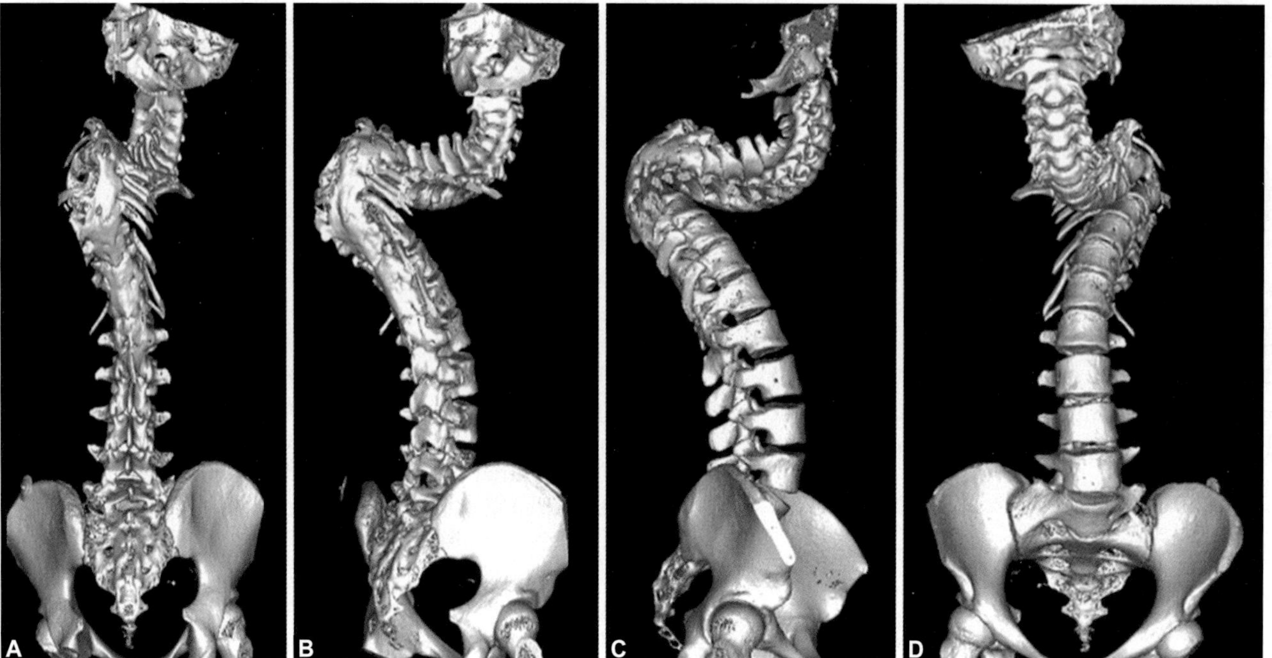

Figs. 8.4A to D: Preoperative three-dimensional computed tomography reconstructions shows severe vertebral wedging and the complexity of the deformity.

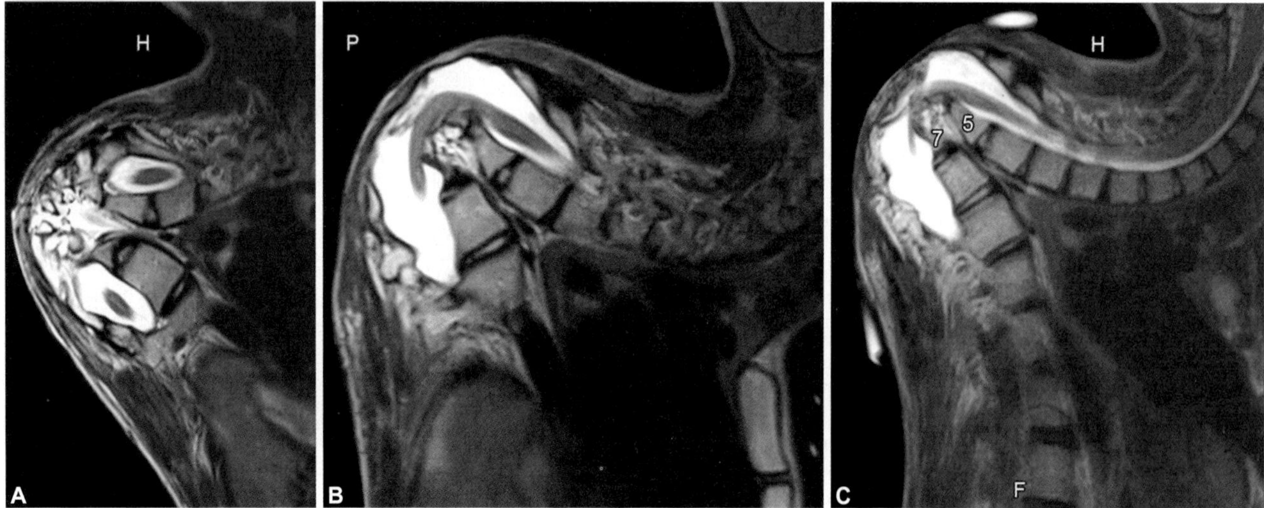

Figs. 8.5A to C: A T2-weighted magnetic resonance imaging demonstrated dural ectasia and spinal cord impingement.

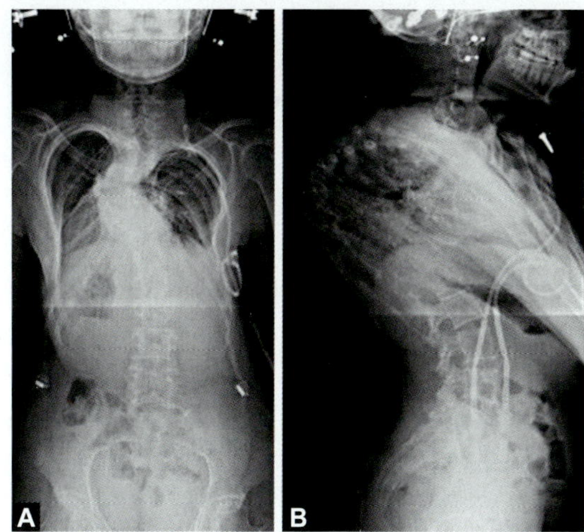

Figs. 8.6A and B: The patient was placed in hanging traction with 20 pounds for over 3 months, with improvements in her radiographic alignment.

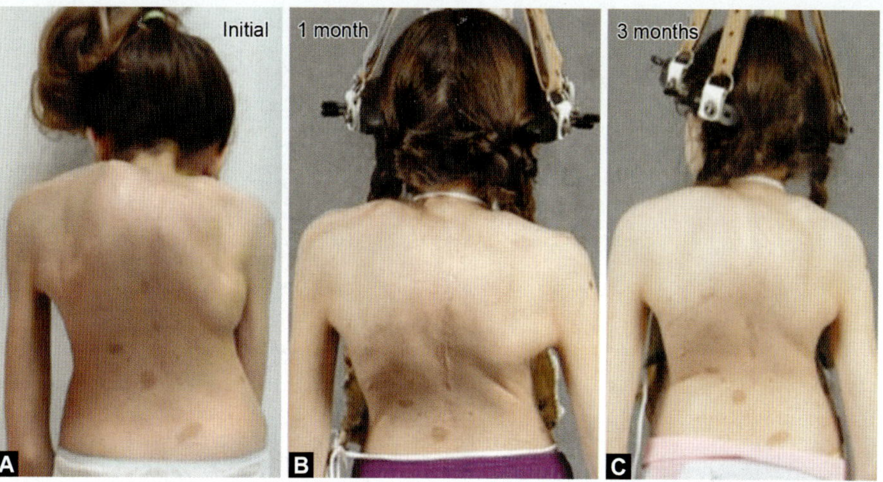

Figs. 8.7A to C: Clinical photos throughout the course of hanging traction with 20 pounds showing improvement in the patient's curve: (A) baseline clinical photo, (B) after 1 month of traction, and (C) after 3 months of traction.

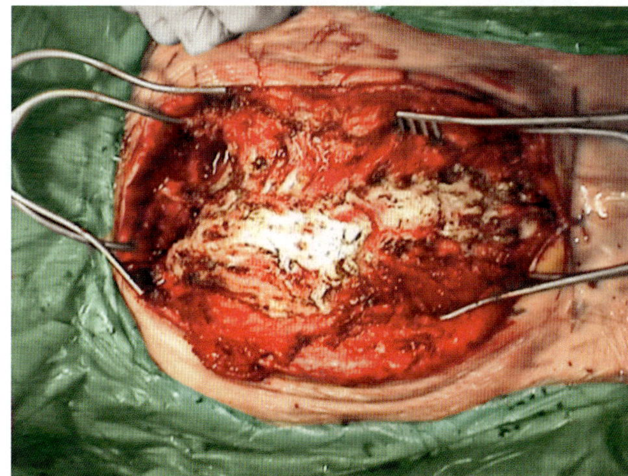

Fig. 8.8: Surgical exposure is wide and thorough, and every effort is made to minimize blood loss during the exposure.

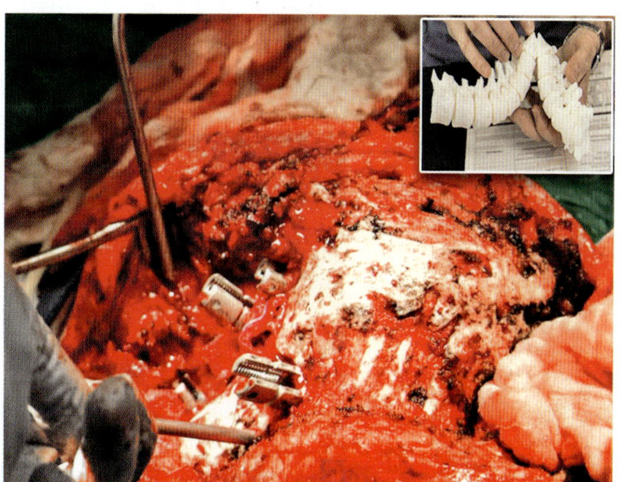

Fig. 8.9: Pedicle screws are placed free-hand, and a three-dimensional resin model of the patient's spine is utilized as a guide throughout this aspect of the procedure.

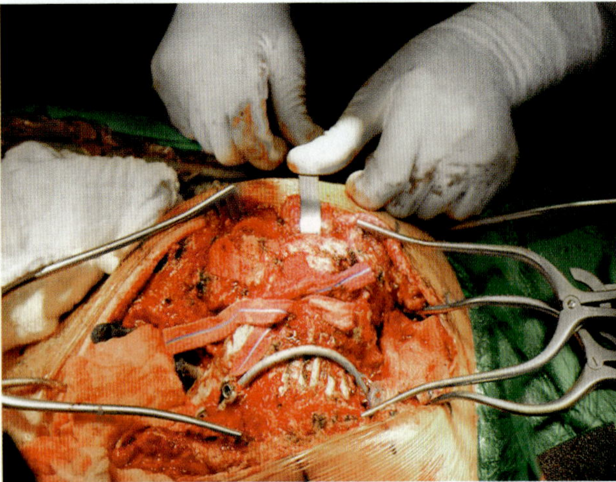

Fig. 8.10: A temporary concave rod is placed for stabilization and the anterior dissection is begun.

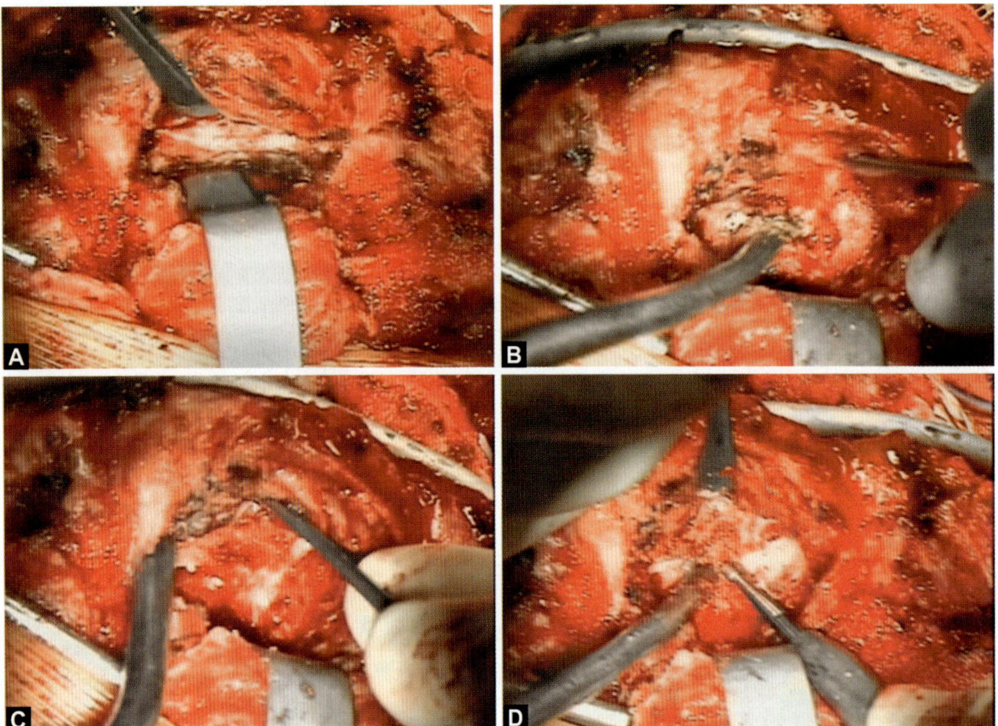

Figs. 8.11A to D: Following stabilization, apical spinal cord exposure, decompression, and vertebral body resection is performed. A high-speed burr is used to remove the bone.

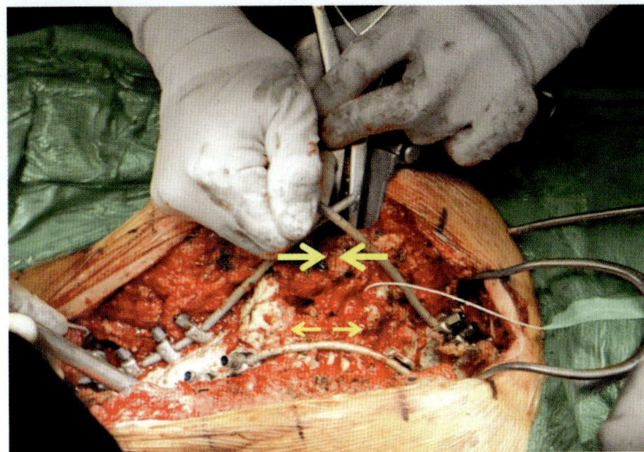

Fig. 8.12: Cantilever correction of the deformity via posterior compression and anterior distraction allows closure through the vertebral column resection.

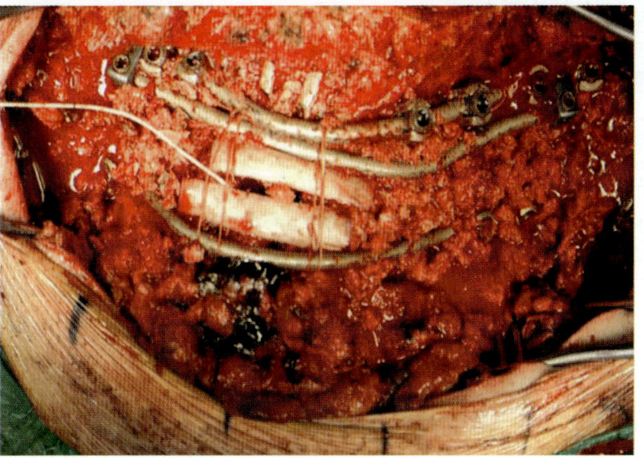

Fig. 8.13: The laminectomy defect of the vertebral column resection is covered with structural rib graft and tied to the contoured rods in situ.

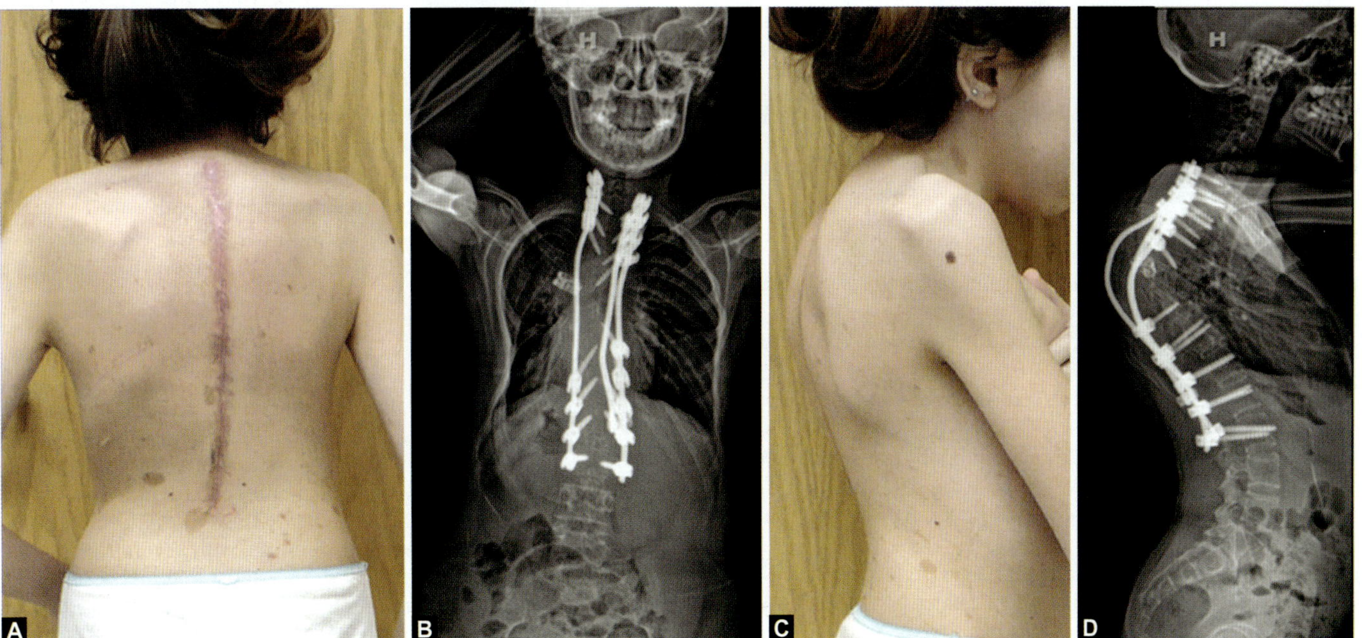

Figs. 8.14A to D: Final postoperative radiographs and clinical images. (A) Posterior clinical image showing a well-healed surgical incision. (B) Anteroposterior radiograph demonstrating significant coronal deformity correction and placement of implants. (C) Lateral clinical image and (D) radiograph illustrating the degree of kyphosis correction achieved.

CONCLUSION

Surgical management of severe spinal deformities is extremely challenging. Historically, a circumferential approach has been the standard of care, and was associated with very high morbidity. Other osteotomy techniques have evolved to allow for dramatic deformity correction and clinical improvement. The posterior-based VCR procedure is a viable, effective tool for the correction of severe spinal deformity in pediatric and adult populations. pVCR allows for significant radiographic deformity correction, as well as improved clinical outcomes and patient satisfaction. Despite being an extremely high-risk procedure, the dramatic improvements that are seen with this technique make it a feasible operation in appropriately selected patients. The treating surgeon's experience level is an important factor in determining the practicality of this advanced technique, but with attentive and reliable spinal cord monitoring, the occurrence of major permanent neurologic deficits can be minimized. The overall complication rate remains high, but a patient undergoing this procedure may still expect improved function and satisfaction postoperatively.

REFERENCES

1. Lenke LG, Newton PO, Sucato DJ, et al. Complications after 147 consecutive vertebral column resections for severe pediatric spinal deformity: a multicenter analysis. Spine (Phila Pa 1976). 2013;38(2):119-32.
2. Suk SI, Chung ER, Kim JH, et al. Posterior vertebral column resection for severe rigid scoliosis. Spine (Phila Pa 1976). 2005;30(14):1682-7.
3. Lenke LG, Sides BA, Koester LA, et al. Vertebral column resection for the treatment of severe spinal deformity. Clin Orthop. 2010;468(3):687-99.
4. MacLennan A. Scoliosis. Br Med J. 1922;2:865-6.
5. Bradford DS. Vertebral column resection. Orthop Trans. 1987;11:502.
6. Enercan M, Ozturk C, Kahraman S, et al. Osteotomies/spinal column resections in adult deformity. Eur Spine J. 2013;22(Suppl 2):S254-64.
7. Suk SI, Kim JH, Kim WJ, et al. Posterior vertebral column resection for severe spinal deformities. Spine (Phila Pa 1976). 2002;27(21):2374-82.
8. Papadopoulos EC, Boachie-Adjei O, Hess WF, et al. Early outcomes and complications of posterior vertebral column resection. Spine J. 2015;15(5):983-91.
9. Calancie B, Harris W, Broton JG, et al. "Threshold-level" multipulse transcranial electrical stimulation of motor cortex for intraoperative monitoring of spinal motor tracts: description of method and comparison to somatosensory evoked potential monitoring. J Neurosurg. 1998;88:457-70.
10. Newton PO, Bastrom TP, Emans JB, et al. Antifibrinolytic agents reduce blood loss during pediatric vertebral column resection procedures. Spine (Phila Pa 1976). 2012;37(23): E1459-63.
11. Hamzaoglu A, Alanay A, Ozturk C, et al. Posterior vertebral column resection in severe spinal deformities: a total of 102 cases. Spine (Phila Pa 1976). 2011;36(5):E340-4.
12. Lenke LG, O'Leary PT, Bridwell KH, et al. Posterior vertebral column resection for severe pediatric deformity minimum two-year follow-up of thirty-five consecutive patients. Spine (Phila Pa 1976). 2009;34(20):2213-21.
13. Gertzbein SD, Harris MB. Wedge osteotomy for the correction of post-traumatic kyphosis. A new technique and a report of three cases. Spine (Phila Pa 1976). 1992;17(3):374-9.
14. Sponseller PD, Jain A, Lenke LG, et al. Vertebral column resection in children with neuromuscular spine deformity. Spine (Phila Pa 1976). 2012;37(11):E655-61.
15. Xie J, Wang Y, Zhao Z, et al. Posterior vertebral column resection for correction of rigid spinal deformity curves greater than 100°. J Neurosurg Spine. 2012;17:540-51.
16. Moon ES, Nanda A, Park JO, et al. Pelvic obliquity in neuromuscular scoliosis: radiologic comparative results of single-stage posterior versus two-stage anterior and posterior approach. Spine (Phila Pa 1976). 2011;36(2):146-52.
17. Auerbach JD, Lenke LG, Bridwell KH, et al. Major complications and comparison between 3-column osteotomy techniques in 105 consecutive spinal deformity procedures. Spine (Phila Pa 1976). 2012;37(14):1198-210.
18. Bullmann V, Schulte TL, Schmidt C, et al. Pulmonary function after anterior double thoracotomy approach versus posterior surgery with costectomies in idiopathic thoracic scoliosis. Eur Spine J. 2013;22(Suppl 2):S164-71.
19. Bumpass DB, Lenke LG, Bridwell KH, et al. Pulmonary function improvement after vertebral column resection for severe spinal deformity. Spine (Phila Pa 1976). 2014;39(7):587-95.
20. O'Neill KR, Lenke LG, Bridwell KH, et al. Factors associated with long-term patient-reported outcomes after three-column osteotomies. Spine J. 2015;15(11):2312-8.
21. Kim SS, Cho BC, Kim JH, et al. Complications of posterior vertebral resection for spinal deformity. Asian Spine J. 2012;6(4):257-65.
22. Cho SK, Bridwell KH, Lenke LG, et al. Major complications in revision adult deformity surgery: risk factors and clinical outcomes with 2- to 7-year follow-up. Spine (Phila Pa 1976). 2012;37(6):489-500.
23. Leatherman KD, Dickerson RA. Two-stage corrective surgery for congenital deformities of the spine. JBJS Br. 1976;61-B(3):324-8.
24. Shimode M, Kojima T, Sowa K. Spinal wedge osteotomy by a single posterior approach for correction of severe and rigid kyphosis or kyphoscoliosis. Spine (Phila Pa 1976). 2002;27(20):2260-7.
25. Wang Y, Xie J, Zhao Z, et al. Preoperative short-term traction prior to posterior vertebral column resection: procedure and role. Eur Spine J. 2016;25(3):687-97.
26. Zhang BB, Zhang T, Tao HR, et al. Neurological complications of thoracic posterior vertebral column resection for severe congenital spinal deformities. Eur Spine J. 2017;26(7):1871-7.
27. Wang Y, Zhang Y, Zhang X, et al. A single posterior approach for multilevel modified vertebral column resection in adults with severe rigid congenital kyphoscoliosis: a retrospective study of 13 cases. Eur Spine J. 2008;17(3):361-72.
28. Wang H, Guo J, Wang S, et al. Instrumentation failure after posterior vertebral column resection in adult spinal deformity. Spine (Phila Pa 1976). 2017;42(7):471-8.

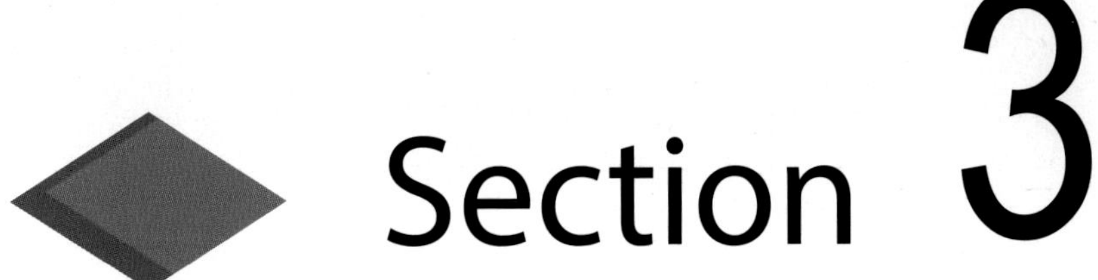

Section 3

Lumbar

- Minimally Invasive Lumbar Decompression for Spinal Stenosis
- Minimal Invasive Transforaminal Interbody Fusion
- Lateral Lumbar Interbody Fusion
- Pedicle Subtraction Osteotomy

CHAPTER

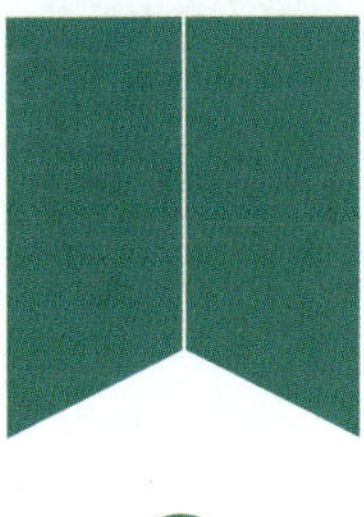

9

Minimally Invasive Lumbar Decompression for Spinal Stenosis

David Kaye, Jacob Borck, D Greg Anderson

ANATOMY

Success with minimally invasive techniques depends on a thorough understanding of both the paraspinal soft tissue anatomy as well as the microscopic anatomy of the spine. Several studies have found that unlike the standard posterior midline approach, minimally invasive approaches may prevent iatrogenic muscle damage and has been demonstrated histologically,[1] enzymatically,[2] electrophysiologically,[3] and clinically to be a less traumatic approach.

One of the goals of minimally invasive spine (MIS) surgery is preservation of the paraspinal musculature. Two paraspinal compartments, each enveloped in its own fascia, exist—(1) the multifidus medially and (2) the longissimus and iliocostalis laterally. In the lumbar region, the multifidus muscle has tendinous origins on the mammillary processes. In the thoracic region, it originates from the transverse processes, while in the cervical region, the multifidus originates at the articular processes of the lower four vertebrae. The fasciculi insert in an upward and medial direction onto the cephalad spinous processes. The multifidus muscle belly covers the medial bony structures of the spine including the spinous processes, lamina, and facet joints. It receives its nerve and blood supply from the medial branches of the dorsal rami and segmental vessels, respectively, which course from the intervertebral foramen along the base of the transverse process and enter the lateral margin of the muscle in the region of the pars intra-articularis. Alternatively, the longissimus and iliocostalis, components of the erector spinae, cover the lateral bony anatomy including the transverse processes.

During an MIS approach, the lumbodorsal fascia, the more robust of the fascial layers, is incised and depending upon the precise trajectory required for a given procedure, a second fascial incision either in the medial or lateral paraspinal compartments is made. Beneath these fascial incisions, the muscles are split, rather than cut, with the use of serial dilators to create a surgical corridor. The interfascial plane between the two deep paraspinal compartments should not be violated as damage to the nerves to the multifidus, running in this interval, can occur.

An understanding of the microscopic anatomy is paramount to a facile MIS procedure. Facet hypertrophy and ligamentum flavum hypertrophy and/or infolding is a major driver of spinal stenosis. The ligamentum is composed of a superficial and deep component. The superficial ligamentum is a light yellow fibrous structure about 2.5–3.5 mm thick that blends into the interspinous ligament and is adjacent to the overlying multifidus. On the cranial lamina, it inserts onto the inferior edge and the anterior inferior surface of the lamina. On the caudal lamina, it inserts onto the posterosuperior surface of the lamina. Conversely, the deep ligament is darker yellow, and only about 1 mm thick, inserting onto the ridge of the cranial lamina between the rougher anteroinferior aspect of the lamina and smoother anterosuperior lamina. On the caudal lamina, it inserts onto the anterosuperior aspect.[4] On the facet joints, the ligamentum extends the length of the joint in the craniocaudal direction and approximately 50% of the width of the joint in the mediolateral plane.

Decompression generally extends from pedicle to pedicle (i.e. for L4-5 decompression, from the pedicle of L4 to the pedicle of L5). Decompression must extend from the top to the bottom of the joint. The rounded contour of the superior articular process (SAP) superiorly must be palpated to ensure the decompression has been carried far enough proximally. Similarly, one must be able to clearly palpate the superomedial aspect of the inferior pedicle to be sure the decompression has been carried far enough distally.

INDICATIONS

The most common surgical indication for spine conditions in the elderly is lumbar spinal stenosis (LSS).[5] Surgery is considered when patients have failed nonoperative management, including physical therapy, nonsteroidal anti-inflammatory medications, and epidural steroid injections. The primary indication for surgery in this setting is neurogenic claudication with concordant findings on advanced imaging [e.g. magnetic resonance imaging (MRI) or computed tomography (CT) myelography].[5,6] Neurogenic claudication typically presents with crampy pain radiating into the legs with erect positioning (i.e. standing or walking) that is relieved with leaning forward or sitting.[7] Alternatively, vascular claudication is generally relieved by halting activity, such as by simply standing still, and typically lacks significant neurologic findings.

The indications for a minimally invasive surgical decompression as opposed to a conventional open procedure are the same. However, MIS, with smaller incisions and less traumatic soft tissue dissection, has the potential to minimize postoperative pain and intraoperative blood loss. Carrying the same risk profile as open decompressive surgery, MIS decompression results in decreased blood loss, shorter hospital stays, and decreased infection rates.[8,9]

TECHNIQUE

Positioning

The patient is positioned prone preferably on a Jackson table with the hip pads positioned just below the iliac crests and the chest pad positioned just below the sternal notch. The abdomen is allowed to hang freely minimizing pressure on the abdominal cavity and helping to prevent excessive epidural bleeding. The table mount for the retractor tube system should be placed just below the hip pads. Before starting, be sure that the fluoroscopy machine can freely pass under the table and that imaging is unencumbered.

Incision Localization

Precise placement of the surgical incision is the first step to a successfully performed MIS procedure. Preoperative X-ray should be carefully interpreted to identify potential transitional anatomy. Preoperative imaging can also be examined to determine the level of the iliac crests which can help with localization. We begin our localization by marking several external landmarks for orientation. After marking the top of the crests, which is usually at the L4-5 intervertebral level, we mark the lateral borders of the spinous processes as well as the PSIS bilaterally. An 18-gauge needle is then placed in a straight up and down direction approximately 2 cm off the lateral edge of the SP at the approximate level of the intervertebral disc. A lateral fluoroscopic image is then obtained to confirm that the intended level can be accessed. Several landmarks are identified on this lateral view. The disc level is the most obvious, but not always the appropriate point to center the incision. Instead, we try to dock the tube at the junction of the inferior aspect of the cranial lamina (i.e. bottom of L4 for an L4-5 decompression) and the spinous process of the same level (i.e. the spinous process of L4 for an L4-5 decompression). On the lateral, this location can be viewed and is frequently found just above the pedicle of the caudal level. After ensuring that the needle is precisely central in the planned incision, the fluoroscopy machine is moved cranially, but remains sterilely prepped into the field. For cases of spinal stenosis where a contralateral decompression will be performed, it is crucial to make the incision laterally enough to be able to access the contralateral side by wanding the tube medially. Therefore, the incision is usually slightly more lateral than it would be for cases of a microdiscectomy. Usually, the incision is approximately 2 cm lateral to the lateral border of the spinous process but that distance increases with increasing body habitus of the patient.

Incision and Docking

We use a 20 mm tube for all MIS procedures so we make a 20 mm incision through the skin. The dissection is then carried through the subcutaneous tissue to the level of the fascia. Electrocautery may be used to coagulate superficial bleeding. The scalpel is then aimed in a medial trajectory in line with the planned trajectory of the tube during decompression and the fascia is incised. By extending the fascial incision proximally and distally beyond the margins of the skin incision, greater mobility of the tube is afforded. After fascial incision, we use a Cobb elevator to gently sweep the muscle off of the spinous process and lamina, also palpating the bony anatomy including the margins of the facet joint. Try not to fall off the facet laterally with blunt dissection as unnecessary bleeding may subsequently be encountered. The initial dilator is then placed through the incision and is used to clearly identify the junction of the spinous process and inferior border of the cranial lamina, appreciating the contours of the lamina and palpating, but not penetrating, the interlaminar space below. The initial dilator is docked on the inferior edge of the lamina at the lamina/SP junction. Serial dilators are sequentially inserted and appropriately sized 20 mm tube in inserted and locked to the table mount. The fluoroscopy machine is brought back to the field and an image is obtained to confirm appropriate placement of the tube. The tube should be all the way down on the bone (the lamina) confirmed by feel and by fluoroscopy as this allows the soft tissue to be pinned between the bone and the tube, facilitating soft tissue clearance for access during the rest of the procedure (Fig. 9.2).

Ipsilateral Decompression

We perform our MIS procedures with the aid of a surgical microscope. At this point, the microscope is bought into the field. Frequently, there will be significant angulation of the tube (Fig. 9.1). To allow for appropriate visualization and for better ergonomics, the table should be rolled to one side or the other and/or in a reverse Trendelenburg or Trendelenburg fashion to lessen the need for awkward surgeon positioning. The goal should be to allow the tube to sit almost upright, rather than in a severely angulated, position.

Bovie electrocautery is used to clear all soft tissue from the underlying bone in the window of the tube. Ideally, the initial tube window should expose the inferior lamina of the cranial level, the upslope of the lamina into the SP, and the beginning of the interlaminar space below. Once cleared of soft tissue, a burr is used to remove bone down to the level of the ligamentum flavum. This sets the depth of the spinal canal for reference throughout the rest of the case. When beginning the bony resection at the inferior aspect of the lamina, the ligamentum flavum will serve as protection for the dura during burring. However, as one moves cranially on the lamina, the ligamentum is absent. More judicious burring is required here to prevent inadvertent dural injury.

Beginning at this inferior laminar margin, use the burr to remove bone, paying attention to the quality of the bone so that the cortical-cancellous-cortical nature of the bone is recognized and utilized to slow burring as the second cortical bone layer is reached. At this level, once the second cortical layer is penetrated, the ligamentum flavum will come into view. Bone may be removed by thinning with a burr until epidural fat is reached at the cranial margin of the ligamentum. More cranial than this, no ligamentum exists and here, we prefer to thin the bone with the burr but to ultimately remove the final pieces with a Kerrison rongeur.

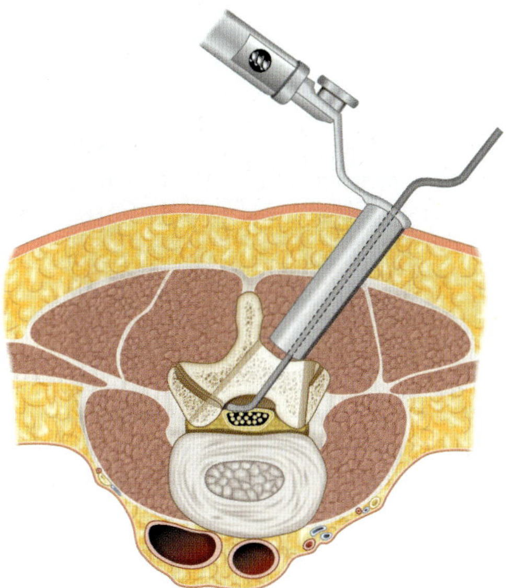

Fig. 9.1: Diagram showing the orientation of the tube to achieve both ipsilateral and contralateral decompression through a unilateral approach.
Source: Link: http://www.texasspineandneurosurgerycenter.com/wp-content/uploads/2012/03/Decompression-Lumbar-Laminectomy.jpg (Medtronic)

Care must be taken not to resect too much bone laterally especially at the level of the pars. We generally try to maintain approximately 1 cm of bone remaining at the pars. To be sure enough bone has been resected to for adequate decompression, but not so much as to destabilize the spine, we use several landmarks. As an external (to the canal) landmark, we resect soft tissue until the fibers of the facet capsule become visible. Initially, the facet capsule serves as the lateral extent of the bony resection. The resection is typically trapezoidal in appearance, wider caudally at the level of the pedicle, and narrower cranially toward the level. We only determine the width of the final decompression once the pedicle is palpated upon canal entry. At the level of the pedicle, the bony resection may proceed until flush with the medial pedicle. However, resection progressively narrows moving cranially on the vertebrae.

Once the ligamentum is visible, the spinal canal may be entered to view the dura with the use of a small curved currete. The currete is used to scrape the undersurface of the lamina, removing the superficial ligamentum flavum from the lamina. The currete may then be turned backward to develop a plan between the ligamentum and dura. Once developed, a Kerrison rongeur may be used to enter the plane and remove the overlying ligamentum. At this point, toward the bottom of the facet joint, the pedicle may be palpated. As already noted, the medial aspect of the pedicle marks the lateral extent of the bony resection inferiorly. Having established this crucial landmark, we can safely resect bone more cranially being sure to leave sufficient bone at the pars. The ligamentum should be removed until the lateral recess and foramen are completely free of compression. For foraminal decompression, the superior aspect of the caudal pedicle and the inferior aspect of the cranial pedicle should be palpated. By hugging the medial aspect of the pedicle (L4 for L4-5 decompression), the exiting nerve root can be appreciated. The exiting nerve root must be protected and the bony overgrowth in the foramen, usually caused by the tip of the SAP, is removed with the use of Kerrison rongeurs. Sometimes, a foraminal Kerrison can be used to better clear the foramen. A ball tipped probe is a useful tool for palpation and assessment of adequate decompression.

Contralateral Decompression

Contralateral decompression starts by first identifying the corridor for entry to the contralateral compartment. We prefer to access the contralateral side beginning at the interspinous ligament at the level of the lamina and SP junction. Frequently, the tube will need to be wanded significantly medially for adequate visualization. After identification of the ligament, we begin removing bone at the lamina/SP

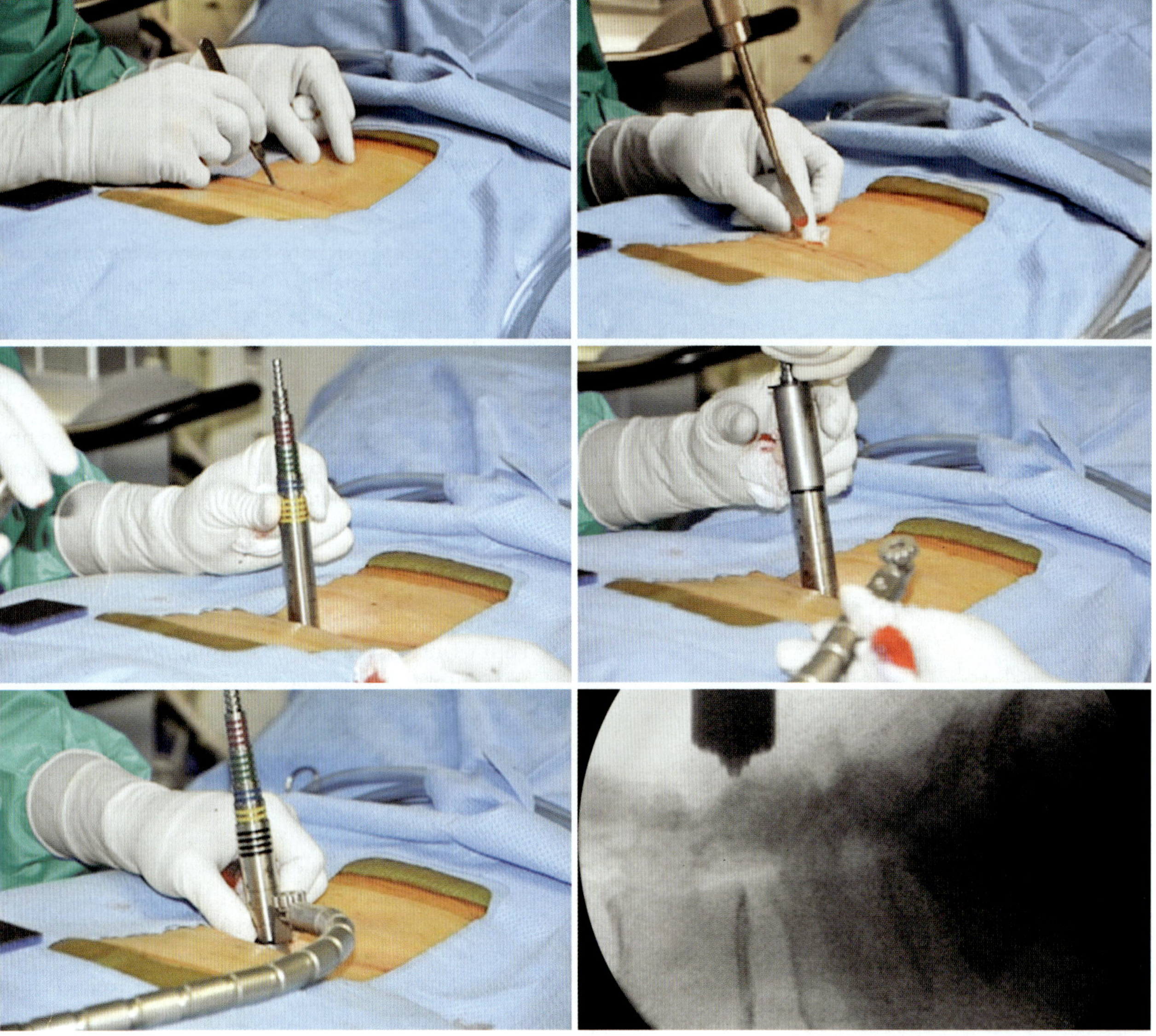

Fig. 9.2: Following needle localization of the targeted disc space, a 2 cm incision is made in line with the needle just off midline. Following fascial incision, a Cobb elevator is used to perform subperiosteal dissection. The tubular retractor is then dilated and positioned taking care to not stray lateral to the facet joint and in line with the disc space on fluoroscopy.

junction moving upward into the SP and contralateral lamina with the use of a burr. An inverted V becomes evident with increasing bony resection at the laminar spinous process junction and once the tip of the V is crossed, resection occurs in the contralateral compartment. As for the ipsilateral side, removal of the SP and lamina progress through a cortical-cancellous-cortical progression. We try to preserve the second cortical layer at the level of the SP to preserve the bony attachments of the paraspinal muscles. However, for increased access, sometimes the inferior half of the SP must be removed in its entirety. If the SP has been completely resected, the paraspinal muscles of the contralateral side will become apparent. The contralateral lamina is then resected with the use of a burr slowing as the second cortical layer is reached. At the inferior half of the lamina, the ligamentum provides a safety net for the contralateral decompression and staying above the ligamentum can prevent dural injury. Once sufficient lamina has been removed, and the underlying ligamentum remains, a curved curette can be used to palpate the undersurface of the lamina and contralateral facet appreciating the rounded contour of the facet compared to the straighter contour of the lamina. The curette is used to release the remaining ligamentum from the remaining bone of the cranial lamina. With the position of the tube, excellent visualization of the contralateral lateral recess is afforded as well as superior visualization of the contralateral foramen. A short ball-tipped probe can be used to help develop a plane between the ligamentum in the contralateral lateral recess and the underlying dura. With gentle downward pressure from the suction to create a plane between the dura and ligamentum, a Kerrison rongeur can be inserted and used to clear the compressive ligamentum. Once the contralateral lateral recess is decompressed, the superior aspect of the pedicle of the level below (L5 for an L4-5 decompression) and the inferior aspect of the pedicle above (L4 for an L4-5 decompression) should be palpated. As for the ipsilateral decompression, inferiorly, the contralateral facet should be removed to be flushed with the medial aspect of the lower pedicle and more bone should be left cranially closer to the pars. The contralateral foramen can be decompressed by staying dorsal to and in the same direction as the exiting nerve root (Fig. 9.2).

Tube Withdrawal and Closure

Most of these MIS decompression cases are performed on the same day of surgery without the use of drains. Therefore, excellent hemostasis must be achieved. Prior to tube withdrawal, bipolar cautery as well as hemostatic agents such as Gelfoam® or Floseal® is used. Bleeding bone edges can be controlled with the use of bone wax. The majority of bleeding occurs in the lateral gutters and once this has been controlled, tube withdrawal begins. We slowly remove the tube under direct visualization being sure achieve complete hemostasis in the soft tissues with the use bipolar cautery. The incision is then closed with #1-vicryl for the fascial closure followed by 2-0 vicryl for subcutaneous closure. We frequently use dermabond for skin closure but monocryl suture can be used alternatively or additionally.

OUTCOMES AND COMPLICATIONS

Surgical management of lumbar spinal stenosis (LSS) has consistently demonstrated improved outcomes compared to nonoperative measures.[10-12] The Maine Lumbar Spine Study showed that by 1 year, 55% of patients treated with surgery experienced significant relief of back and leg pain compared to only 28% of those managed nonoperatively.[11] By 10 years, patients undergoing surgery continued to show superiority in terms of leg pain and back related functional status.[12]

Eight-year data from the spine patient outcomes research trial (SPORT) trial similarly documents continued improvement of surgical versus nonsurgical care for the management of spinal stenosis.[10] The SPORT trial is a multicenter prospective trial, conducted across 11 states at 13 medical centers, comparing the results of surgical versus nonsurgical management of lumbar spine conditions. The trial includes both a randomized cohort [randomized controlled trial (RCT)] and a concurrent observational cohort [observational study (OBS)] with 654 patients enrolled in the spinal stenosis cohort (289 in the RCT and 365 in the OBS) and approximately 55% of patients available for an 8-year follow-up. In the as-treated analysis combining the RCT and OBS cohorts, at 8 years, surgically treated patients experienced significantly greater improvement in pain, function, satisfaction, and self-rated progress.[10]

However, a subset of patients undergoing operative management of LSS is unsatisfied with their outcomes with as many as 40% experiencing chronic lower back pain. Some have attributed these residual symptoms to the invasiveness of the open approach, as prolonged muscle retraction can lead to muscle atrophy,[13] as confirmed by radiographic (CT) and [electromyography (EMG)] studies.[14]

Minimally invasive decompression (MID) has been introduced in part to address these concerns. A recent meta-analysis found that the satisfaction rate for MID was 84% compared to 75.4% for open laminectomy.[8] Other benefits of the MIS approach include decreased blood loss, decreased postoperative pain scores, and shortened hospital stays. Studies have been equivocal regarding operative time which likely reflects the learning curve associated with procedure.[8]

Complications, including cerebrospinal fluid (CSF) leaks, wound infection, and medical complications [pneumonia, myocardial infarction (MI), venous thromboembolism (VTE), etc.] are equivalent between open and MIS approaches. However, reoperation rates are lower for the MIS approach (1.6 vs. 5.8%).[8]

Discussion of MIS needs to be expanded in terms of outcomes.

Complications need to be expanded.

CASE PRESENTATION

A 61-year-old healthy, active male presents with over 1 year of right greater than left lower extremity pain radiating from the buttocks to the anterior thigh and posterolateral thigh and calf. Pain is claudicatory in nature and has been refractory to conservative treatment including nonsteroidal anti-inflammatory drugs (NSAIDs), physical therapy, and epidural steroid injections. MRI demonstrated moderate stenosis especially in the lateral recess at L3-4 and L4-5 (Figs. 9.3A and B). Given the patient's active lifestyle, he was offered a less invasive approach for surgical management. A two-level MIS decompression was performed utilizing a tubular retractor through a unilateral approach. A slightly longer incision is utilized for a two-level approach with care taken to wand under fluoroscopic guidance to

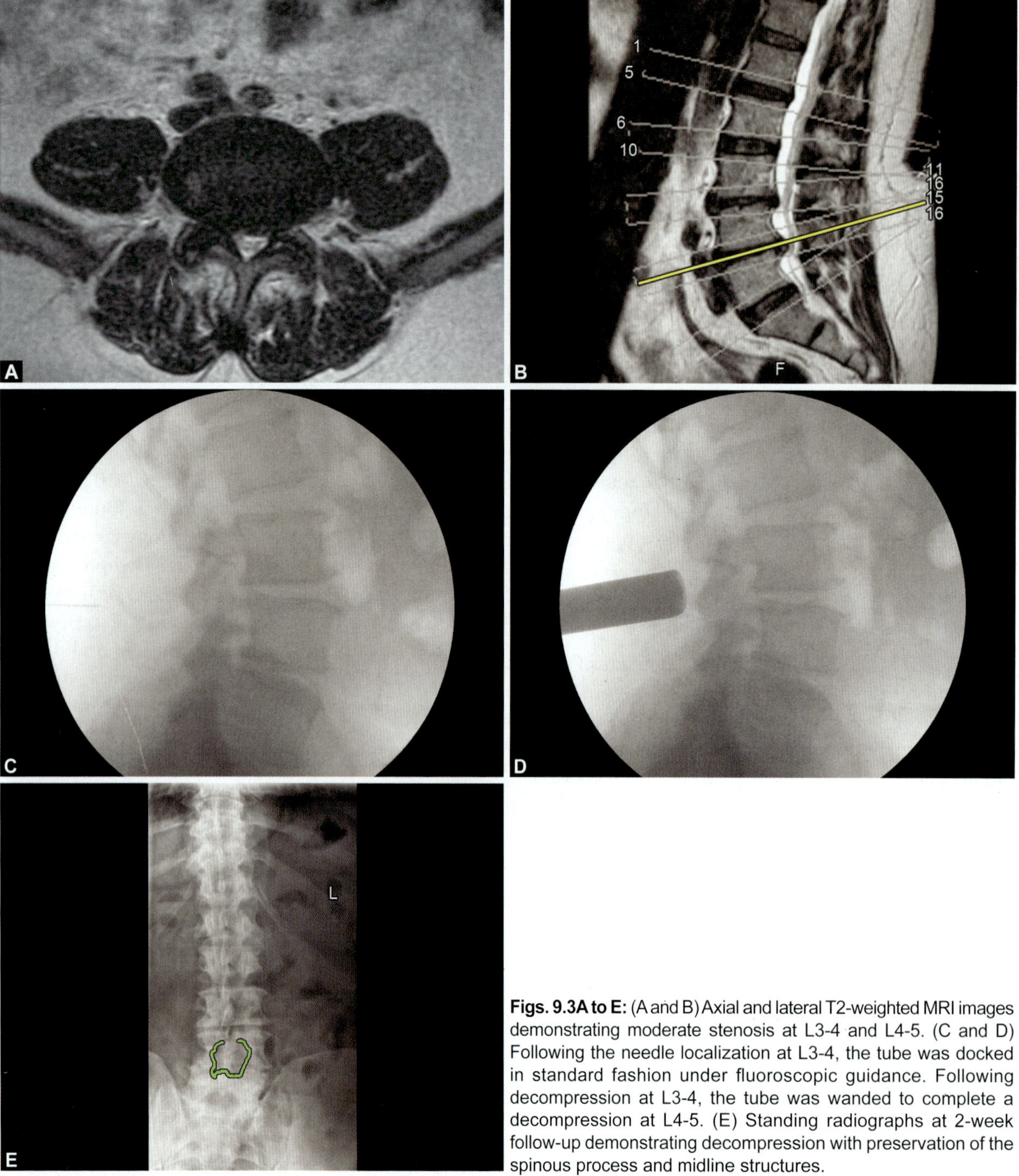

Figs. 9.3A to E: (A and B) Axial and lateral T2-weighted MRI images demonstrating moderate stenosis at L3-4 and L4-5. (C and D) Following the needle localization at L3-4, the tube was docked in standard fashion under fluoroscopic guidance. Following decompression at L3-4, the tube was wanded to complete a decompression at L4-5. (E) Standing radiographs at 2-week follow-up demonstrating decompression with preservation of the spinous process and midline structures.

the appropriate levels (Figs. 9.3C to E). Following the surgery, the patient was kept overnight for monitoring and mobilization with physical therapy. He was discharged the following morning with complete relief of his leg pain and minimal back discomfort. At the 2-week follow-up appointment, the patient was eager to return to activities and radiographs demonstrated a complete decompression with no evidence of instability (Figs. 9.4A and B).

Case Presentation

Anand Segar, Tyler Kreitz

Minimally Invasive Lumbar Decompression for Stenosis

A 66-year-old gentleman presented with symptoms of neurogenic claudication. Examination was unremarkable except for bilateral L5 weakness. A lumbar MRI demonstrated stenosis at L4-5 and a central disc protrusion causing stenosis at L5-S1 (Figs. 9.5A and B).

He underwent a minimally invasive L4-S1 decompression sparing the posterior tension band and spinous process. Preoperative X-rays show spondylosis without the presence of a spondylolisthesis.

Postoperative axial CT showed preservation of the tip of the spinous process and adequate bony decompression (Fig. 9.6). Postoperative anteroposterior (AP) and flexion X-rays showed no iatrogenic instability (Figs. 9.7A and B).

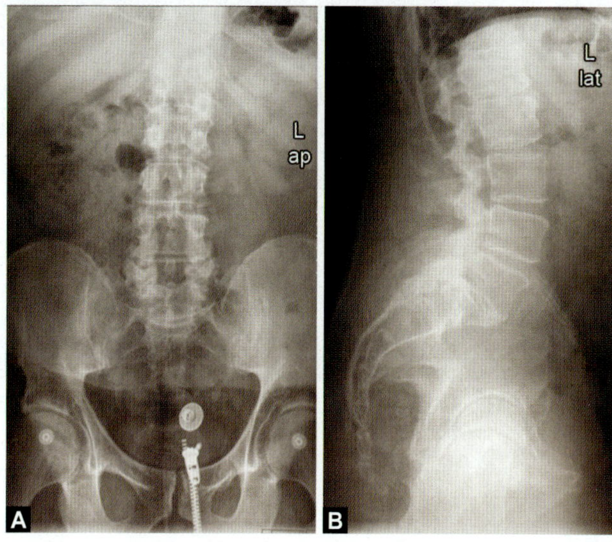

Figs. 9.4A and B: (A) Preoperative anteroposterior X-ray. (B) Preoperative lateral X-ray.

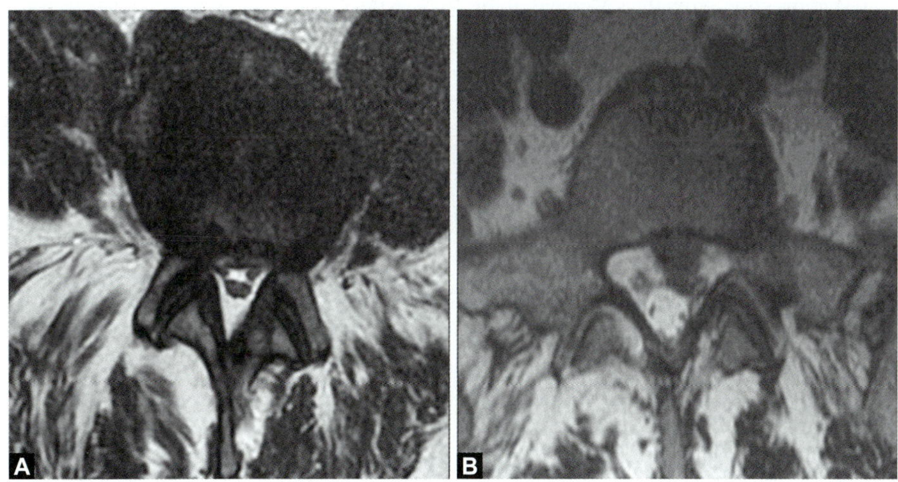

Figs. 9.5A and B: (A) Preopertive T2-weighted axial MRI scan at L4/5 disc space. (B) Preopertive T2-weighted axial MRI scan at L5/S1 disc space.

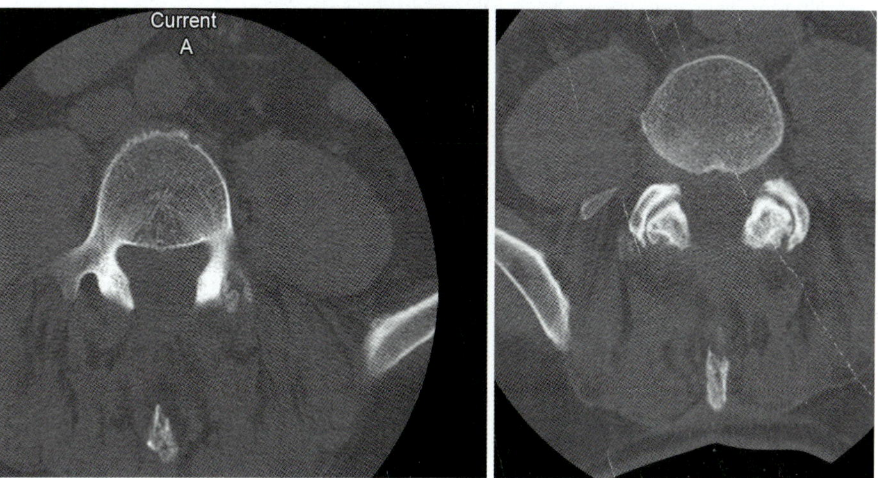

Fig. 9.6: Postoperative axial CT.

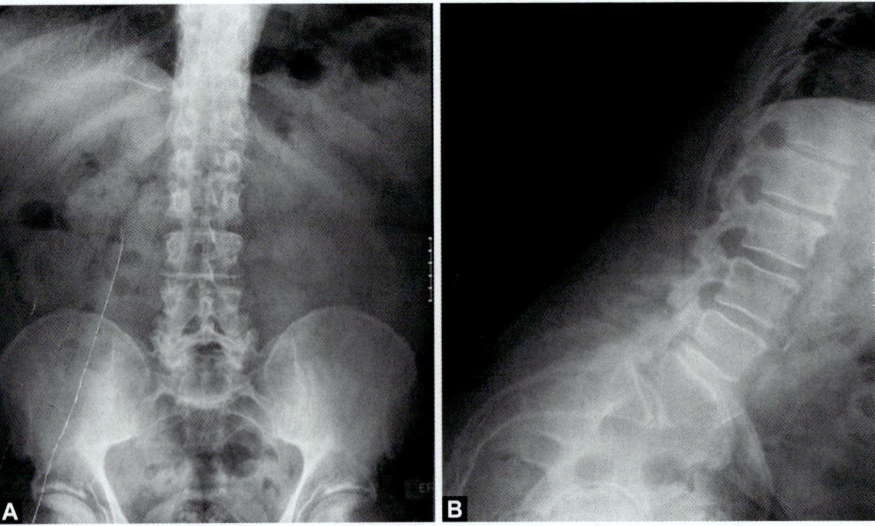

Figs. 9.7A and B: (A) Postoperative anteroposterior X-ray. (B) Postoperative flexion X-ray. *Courtesy:* Dr Alexander R Vaccaro.

REFERENCES

1. Weber BR, Grob D, Dvorak J, et al. Posterior surgical approach to the lumbar spine and its effect on the multifidus muscle. Spine. 1997;22:1765-72.
2. Kawaguchi Y, Matsui H, Tsuji H. Changes in serum creatine phosphokinase MM isoenzyme after lumbar spine surgery. Spine. 1997;22:1018-23.
3. Kramer M, Katzmaier P, Eisele R, et al. Surface electromyography-verified muscular damage associated with the open dorsal approach to the lumbar spine. Eur Spine J. 2001;10:414-20.
4. Olszewski AD, Yaszemski MJ, White AA 3rd. The anatomy of the human lumbar ligamentum flavum. New observations and their clinical importance. Spine. 1996;21:2307-12.
5. Atlas SJ, Keller RB, Robson D, et al. Surgical and nonsurgical management of lumbar spinal stenosis: four-year outcomes from the Maine Lumbar Spine Study. Spine. 2000;25(5):556-62.
6. Barz T, Melloh M, Staub LP, et al. Nerve root sedimentation sign: evaluation of a new radiological sign in lumbar spinal stenosis. Spine. 2010;35(8):892-7.
7. Kalichman L, Cole R, Kim DH, et al. Spinal stenosis prevalence association with symptoms: the Framingham Study. Spine J. 2009;9(7):545-50.
8. Phan K, Mobbs RJ. Minimally invasive versus open laminectomy for lumbar stenosis: a systematic review and meta-analysis. Spine. 2016;41(2):E91-100.
9. Kulkarni AG, Patel RS, Dutta S. Does minimally invasive spine surgery minimize surgical site infections? Asian Spine J. 2016;10(6):1000-6.
10. Lurie JD, Tosteson TD, Tosteson A, et al. Long-term outcomes of lumbar spinal stenosis: eight-year results of the Spine Patient Outcomes Research Trial (SPORT). Spine. 2015;40(2):63-76.
11. Atlas SJ, Deyo RA, Keller RB, et al. The Maine Lumbar Spine Study, Part III: 1-year outcomes of surgical and nonsurgical management of lumbar spinal stenosis. Spine (Phila Pa 1976). 1996;21(15):1787-95.
12. Atlas SJ, Keller RB, Wu YA, et al. Long-term outcomes of surgical and nonsurgical management of lumbar spinal stenosis: 8 to 10 year results from the Maine lumbar spine study. Spine (Phila Pa 1976). 2005;30(8):936-43.
13. Datta G, Gnanalingham KK, Peterson D, et al. Back pain and disability after lumbar laminectomy: is there a relationship to muscle retraction? Neurosurg. 2004;54:1413-20.
14. See DH, Kraft GH. Electromyography in paraspinal muscles following surgery for root compression. Arch Phys Med Rehabilit. 1975;56:80-3.

CHAPTER

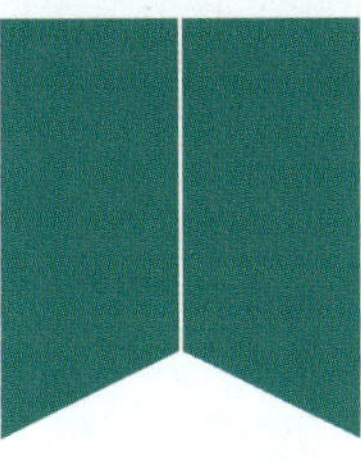

10

Minimal Invasive Transforaminal Interbody Fusion

Tyler Kreitz, David Kaye, Mark Kurd

ANATOMY

The lumbar paraspinal muscles are responsible for maintaining posture and protecting the integrity of intervertebral discs, facet joints, and adjacent ligaments. Minimally invasive surgical (MIS) principles take advantage of intramuscular planes to avoid damage to the osseo-tendinous attachment of the paraspinal musculature, specifically the multifidus and erector spinae, and maintain the integrity of the dorsolumbar fascia.[1-3] MIS techniques minimize the surgical corridor, operative blood loss, perioperative morbidity, and expedite recovery without affecting outcomes compared to open procedures.[4-7] Techniques involve fluoroscopic localization, definition of intramuscular planes, and use of tubular retractors allowing for gentle muscle retraction rather than resection and elevation to visualize bony anatomy. Transforaminal lumbar interbody fusion (TLIF) relies on resection of the superior articular process of the caudal vertebrae and inferior articular process of the cephalad vertebrae to provide safe access to the intervertebral disc. This anatomic safe zone, also known as Kambin's triangle, is formed by the caudal pedicle, traversing, and exiting nerve root. Resection of the intervertebral disc and insertion of an interbody device allows for restoration of disc space height, lumbar lordosis, and both direct and indirect decompression of the bilateral nerve roots.

INDICATIONS

Indications for MIS TLIF mirror those of open TLIF and are highly dependent on a surgeons experience and comfort with MIS techniques. Indications include:

- Degenerative spondylolisthesis
- Grade I and II isthmic spondylolisthesis
- Degenerative scoliosis
- Recurrent disc herniation
- Severe foraminal stenosis not amenable to decompression alone
- Pseudarthrosis.

All patients should have cross-sectional imaging demonstrating nerve root compression and corresponding neurologic symptoms that are refractory to a course of appropriate nonoperative management. Nonoperative management may include anti-inflammatory medications, physical therapy, and epidural steroid injections. Concomitant conditions mimicking radiculopathy must be excluded, including forms of central and peripheral neuropathy. Progressive neurologic symptoms including worsening motor symptoms and signs of cauda equine syndrome may necessitate expedited operative intervention.

CONTRAINDICATIONS

The only absolute contraindication for MIS TLIF is a conjoined nerve root over the transforaminal discectomy window. This finding is rare and may be seen on preoperative MRI evaluation. Patients with high-grade spondylolisthesis may be better treated via an open approach but ultimately depends on surgeons experience with MIS techniques. In patients with a BMI greater than 40, the working distance of the tubular retractor system increases and morbid obesity may be a relative contraindication to

MIS techniques. Although not an absolute contraindication, performing a MIS TLIF at more than two adjacent levels can also be challenging.

TECHNIQUE

Instruments

- Open Jackson table
- Intraoperative fluoroscopy
- Surgical loupes or microscope
- Tube retractor system
- Minimally invasive surgical instrument set (bayoneted instruments)
- High-speed burr
- Cannulated pedicle screws with guide wires, Jamshidi needles, rod passer
- Disc prep instruments
- Interbody device
- Bone allograft material.

Positioning

- The patient is placed prone on an open Jackson frame with a platform for hip extension allowing for restoration of lumbar lordosis.
- Bony prominences including the anterior superior iliac spines (ASIS) are well padded.
- Arms are placed on arm boards with shoulders abducted and externally rotated and elbows flexed to approximately 90°.
- The patient is prepped and draped in sterile fashion.

Incision and Exposure

- A guide wire is used under anterior-posterior (AP) fluoroscopy to mark two horizontal lines bisecting the midpoint of the target cephalad and caudad pedicles. A modified Ferguson or "inlet and outlet" view may be necessary to obtain a perfect AP of each pedicle and cephalad endplate depending on the vertebral level and degree of lumbar lordosis.
- A vertical line is made along the patients' midline in-line with the spinous processes.
- Two vertical lines are then made along the lateral border of the left and right pedicles to be included in the construct.
- *Pearl: Perfect AP and lateral fluoroscopic images are critical to accurate incision placement and instrumentation. Ferguson or "inlet" and "outlet" views may be necessary to obtain the AP image. The degree of c-arm rotation should be noted for each vertebra so that it may be reproduced. An experienced fluoroscopic technician can be very helpful with this step. If appropriate fluoroscopic images are unable to be obtained, MIS TLIF may be converted to open procedure.*
- The side of the most significant leg pain is chosen for exposure and interbody insertion. A local nerve block agent (e.g., bupivacaine hydrochloride and epinephrine) may be used to infiltrate the skin, subcutaneous tissue, and paraspinal musculature.
- A vertical skin incision is made roughly 2 cm lateral to the lateral border of the pedicles previously marked.
- The incision is carried to and through the lumbodorsal fascia and muscle epimysium.
- *Pearl: The incision may need to be farther from midline in larger patients to adequately access the contralateral disc space.*

Guide Wire Placement

- A perfect AP view of the vertebral body is obtained. This includes a crisp superior endplate and a spinous process that bisects the pedicles. Alternatively, two c-arms can be used to obtain AP and lateral images simultaneously.
- A Jamshidi needle is placed through the incision to the lateral midpoint of the pedicle at the 3 o'clock (right) and 9 o'clock (left) position. The needle can be used to palpate the transverse process and then "walked" medially to the appropriate starting point. The needle tip is seated a few millimeters into the bone using a mallet and position again confirmed on AP fluoroscopy.
- The Jamshidi is further impacted into the pedicle parallel to the endplate shadow with roughly 10° medial angulation. It is impacted roughly 20 mm, past the pedicle isthmus. Resistance may be encountered at the physeal scar.
- Fluoroscopy is used to assess the position of the needle tip, which lies approximately one-half to two-thirds of the distance (from medial to lateral) across the pedicle and to ensure the Jamshidi does not violate the medial wall of the pedicle.
- A guide wire is placed through the Jamshidi and advanced an additional 15 mm. The Jamshidi is removed leaving the guide wire in place.
- This process is then repeated for each pedicle (Fig. 10.1).

Tubular Retractor Placement

- The c-arm is moved to obtain lateral images.
- The starting dilator is placed through the same incision on the caudal aspect of the cephalad lamina, confirmed on lateral fluoroscopy.
- Sequential dilators are placed to accept a 20–26 mm tubular retractor. Lateral X-ray is used to confirm collinearity with the target disc space.
- The tubular retractor is secured to the Jackson frame.

Laminectomy/Facetectomy

- A microscope or loupe magnification is used for the decompression, disc exposure, and interbody preparation. Electrocautery is used to remove the facet capsule and remaining soft tissue to fully expose the ipsilateral lamina, pars, and facet joint.

- A side-cutting burr is then used to perform an ipsilateral laminotomy up to the insertion of the ligamentum flavum. If a bilateral direct decompression is required, a burr can be used to perform a sublaminar contralateral decompression and a Kerrison can be used to excise the contralateral ligamentum flavum and decompress the contralateral lateral recess.
- A burr is used to osteotomize the pars, in line with the inferior endplate of the cephalad vertebrae, and resect the inferior articular process of the cephalad level.
- An osteotome, burr, or Kerrison rongeur is used to resect the superior articular facet until flush with the caudal pedicle. Similar to an open TLIF, the pedicle should be adequately skeletonized. Bone fragments are saved for use in interbody fusion.
- The ligamentum flavum is resected using a Kerrison rongeur from the cephalad and caudal lamina to reveal the dural sac, traversing nerve root and intervertebral disc within Kambin's triangle.
- Epidural veins should be cauterized using bipolar electrocautery.
- The traversing nerve may be gently retracted with a nerve root retractor by an assistant if necessary.
- The disc space is accessed through a window bordered medially by the dural sac and traversing nerve root, cephalad by the exiting nerve root, and caudad by the pedicle.
- *Pearl: In patients with severe stenosis or those with previous epidural steroid injection, the dura may be adhered to the ligamentum flavum, predisposing to a dural tear. Care must also be taken when releasing the cephalad insertion of the ligamentum. The dura may be adhered to the undersurface of the cephalad lamina, or where the ligamentum flavum becomes confluent with the facet capsule.*

Discectomy

- The annulus fibrosis is incised creating a rectangular window using a scalpel.
- A pituitary is used to remove disc fragments until a shaver may be placed.
- Sequential use of shavers, pituitary, and Kerrison rongeur is used to remove the intervertebral disc.
- A curette is then used to remove the cartilaginous endplates to provide fully denuded surfaces confirming a thorough discectomy. A burr may be used to puncture the endplate to promote hematopoietic elements into the fusion mass. Though care should be taken to avoid significant endplate violation, which may result in subsidence of the interbody device.
- Lateral fluoroscopy may be used to determine the depth of instrumentation into the disc space and reduce the chance of anterior annulus penetration, risking significant vascular injury.
- The disc space is then irrigated.
- *Pearl: Care should be taken to protect the traversing and exiting nerve root during disc space preparation and interbody insertion. The traversing nerve root is protected using a D'Errico or similar nerve root retractor.*

Interbody Device Insertion

- The excavated disc space is sized for the appropriate interbody device using trial sizers.
- Bone graft is morselized and packed within the interbody cage. Generally 30–45 cc allograft cancellous chips are necessary to augment the autograft bone. A funnel may be used to impact the allograft material into the disc space. The cage is then placed, positioned based on the pathology. Asymmetric for scoliosis, posterior for better foraminal decompression, ventral for increased lordosis, etc. The remainder of the disc space is impacted with morselized allograft.
- *Pearl: Solid interbody fusion is critical to MIS TLIF procedures compared to open TLIF, which may obtain a more reliable posterolateral fusion in addition to interbody fusion. A gentle palpation and proper visualization ensures the absence of exiting and traversing nerve root compression at the conclusion of interbody insertion and bone grafting.*

Pedicle Screw Placement

- Using lateral fluoroscopy, a tap is placed over each guide wire followed by placement of the pedicle screw.
- Lateral fluoroscopy is used to ensure safe depth of instrumentation within the pedicle.
- The pedicle tap or screws may be tested using electromyography (EMG) neuromonitoring. This step is repeated for each pedicle.
- Each rod is then passed through the tulip heads and locked into place using torqued set screws.
- Final AP and lateral fluoroscopy are used to confirm appropriate positioning of the fusion construct (Figs. 10.1A to F).
- *Pearl: When preparing for pedicle screw placement, the guide wire should always be held when passing instruments to prevent inadvertent advancement or removal of the guide wire.*

Closure

- The wound is then irrigated. Bleeding is controlled using electrocautery.
- The fascia, subcutaneous tissue, and skin are closed in multiple layers. A sterile dressing is placed.

Postoperative Protocol

Early ambulation on postoperative day 0 is encouraged. Patients are typically discharged postoperative day 1 or 2. The routine use of segmental compression devices is recommended for the prevention of deep vein thrombosis. The authors recommend no heavy lifting, twisting, or bending for up to 12 weeks or until fusion is demonstrated.

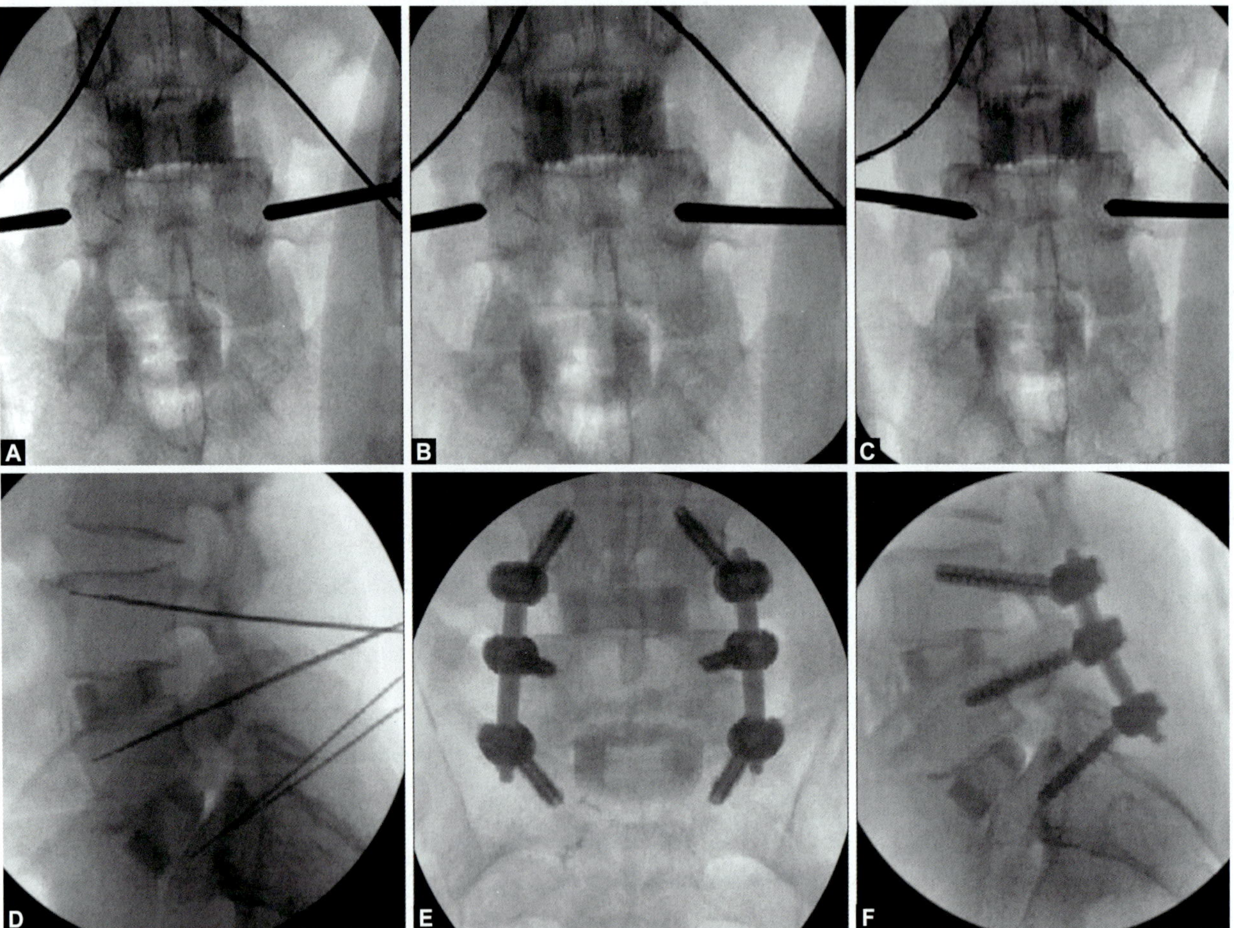

Figs. 10.1A to F: Following anterior interbody grafting at L4-5 and L5-S1, the L4 pedicles are cannulated and guide wires placed. A perfect anterior-posterior (AP) of the L5 pedicle is obtained and Jamshidi needles are positioned at the 9 and 3 o'clock positions on the pedicle (A). Each Jamshidi needle is advanced 20 mm taking care not to breach past the medial pedicle (B and C). Following guide wire placement on AP fluoroscopy, lateral fluoroscopy is obtained to confirm appropriate guide wire positioning (D). Following this, pedicles are tapped and screws are placed over the guide wires. This was followed by a final rod placement (E and F).

OUTCOMES

Several studies have demonstrated short-term benefits of MIS techniques including: decreased intraoperative blood loss, improved postoperative pain control, and reduced hospital length of stay.[4-8] A systematic review of 966 patients undergoing MIS TLIF compared to 863 undergoing open TLIF by Phan et al.[8] demonstrated decreased blood loss, lower infection rates (1.2 vs 4.6%), lower visual analog score (VAS) back, and Oswestry disability index (ODI) scores in the MIS patients. There was no difference in operating time between MIS and open procedures.[8] Fewer studies have evaluated the long-term outcomes of MIS procedures. One retrospective study by Seng et al.[6] evaluated 5-year clinical and radiographic outcomes of 40 patients undergoing MIS TLIF matched to an open cohort. They demonstrated similar fusion rates (97.5%), complication, and reoperation rates at 5 years, with MIS procedures demonstrating significantly lower blood loss (127 vs 405 mL) and hospital length of stay (3.6 vs 5.9 days).[6] MIS techniques may also reduce healthcare costs. A prospective cost analysis by Singh et al.[9] compared outcomes and hospital costs of 33 patients undergoing MIS compared to 33 open TLIF procedures. They demonstrated shorter operative time (115 vs 186 min), reduced length of stay (2.3 vs 2.9 days), and lower direct hospital costs ($19,512 vs $23,550) for the MIS group.[9] Multiple studies have demonstrated reduced blood loss, improved pain control, and reduced hospital length of stay in patients undergoing MIS TLIF compared to open procedures. Further high-quality studies are necessary to evaluate the long-term outcomes of MIS TLIF.

The learning curve associated with MIS techniques is a common concern among surgeons.[10-12] One meta-analysis demonstrated an intraoperative adverse event rate of 11% for a surgeon's first 30 MIS decompressions, decreasing to less than 1% thereafter. The most common adverse event was incidental durotomy. Several single institution studies have demonstrated a higher complication rate, longer OR time, and greater intraoperative blood loss during a surgeon's first 30–40 MIS TLIF procedures.[13-15] Another retrospective review of a single surgeons experience demonstrated no difference in perioperative complications during initial 30 MIS TLIF procedures, with reduced operative time and blood loss for those performed thereafter.[13] Surgeons should be aware of the learning curve associated with MIS techniques. Available data suggests this period occurs during a surgeon's first 30 MIS cases.[11,13-15] A novice surgeon should be cautious and meticulous as their MIS techniques are refined.

Use of routine intraoperative fluoroscopy is not without risk. Fluoroscopically guided pedicle screw placement exposes surgeons to 10–12 times the dose of radiation compared to nonfluoroscopically aided musculoskeletal procedures. Spine surgeons regularly performing routine MIS surgery may be at a higher risk of fatal cancer.[16] A surgeon's experience and familiarity with MIS techniques is likely to reduce the extent of fluoroscopic exposure necessary for MIS procedures, thereby reducing associated exposure risks.

COMPLICATIONS

- Dural tear
- Nerve root injury
- Infection
- Pseudarthrosis
- Hardware malposition
- Medical complications.

CORTICAL SCREWS

In 2009, Santoni et al. introduced the concept of cortical screw placement to improve screw purchase and address loosening rates in patients with poor bone quality.[17] Cortical bone tract screws enhance cortical purchase through a laterally directed trajectory in the transverse plane and a superiorly directed tract in the sagittal plane. Traditional pedicle screws obtain the majority of their fixation in the dense cortical bone of the pedicle; but as much as 20–40% of their purchase occurs within trabecular bone of the vertebral body. In patients with osteoporosis, trabecular bone is compromised, leading to increased rates of loosening and screw cut-out.[18-20] A cortical screw technique was developed to improve bone purchase in patients with poor bone quality. Several in vivo and ex vivo studies have demonstrated increased insertional torque,[21,22] pullout strength,[17] and cortical screw toggle strength under cyclic loading[23] compared to traditional pedicle screws.

Cortical Screw Technique

- Use of fluoroscopic guidance is recommended.
- The starting point for screw insertion is marked with a burr using AP fluoroscopy. The point is located approximately 1 mm inferior to the caudal border of the transverse process and center of the superior articular process and 1 mm from the lateral edge of the pars for L1 in a medial to lateral plane. This point moves sequentially farther from the pars edge in more caudal vertebrae. Fluoroscopy may be used to confirm these relative landmarks with start point along the 5 or 7 o'clock position of the left and right pedicle silhouette.
- The cortical screw tract is drilled using a bit sized to the minor diameter of the intended screw. The drill tract follows a 10° medial to lateral and 25° caudocephalad trajectory aiming for the 11-or-1 o'clock direction on the left or right pedicle. On a lateral fluoroscopic image, the drill trajectory engages the inferior half of the pedicle and ends at the posterior third of the vertebral body (Figs. 10.2A and B).
- A ball tip probe is used to ensure that the medial or inferior pedicle wall has not been violated requiring reposition of the cortical tract. Violation of the lateral vertebral wall rarely causes neurovascular injury and may safely accept screw placement if redirection is not possible.
- Line to line tapping is recommended, i.e. a 5.5 mm tap is used for a 5.5 mm screw.
- Preferred screw length is 35–40 mm, engaging the posterior third to half of the vertebral body.

Complications specific to cortical screw placement include pars and pedicle fractures. Iatrogenic pars fracture requires conversion to traditional pedicle screw fixation. There are no specific indications for cortical over pedicle screws, but they may offer improved bone purchase and reduced cut out rates in patients with poor bone quality. The use of cortical screws in minimally invasive procedures is also gaining acceptance. The medial to lateral tract requires less dissection and a narrower field compared to traditional pedicle screws. A review of 202 patients undergoing cortical tract lumbar screws demonstrated a low rate of facet joint violation (11.8%) by computerized tomography (CT) scan evaluation, compared to published rates of 25–100% for traditional pedicle screws.[24] A facet joint violation may result in increased mechanical instability at adjacent segments, precluding to adjacent segment disease.[25,26] A retrospective review of patients undergoing cortical screw placement demonstrated a reduced rate of adjacent segment disease (3.2 vs 11%), compared to pedicle screws.[27] The facet sparing nature of cortical screws may also provide benefit

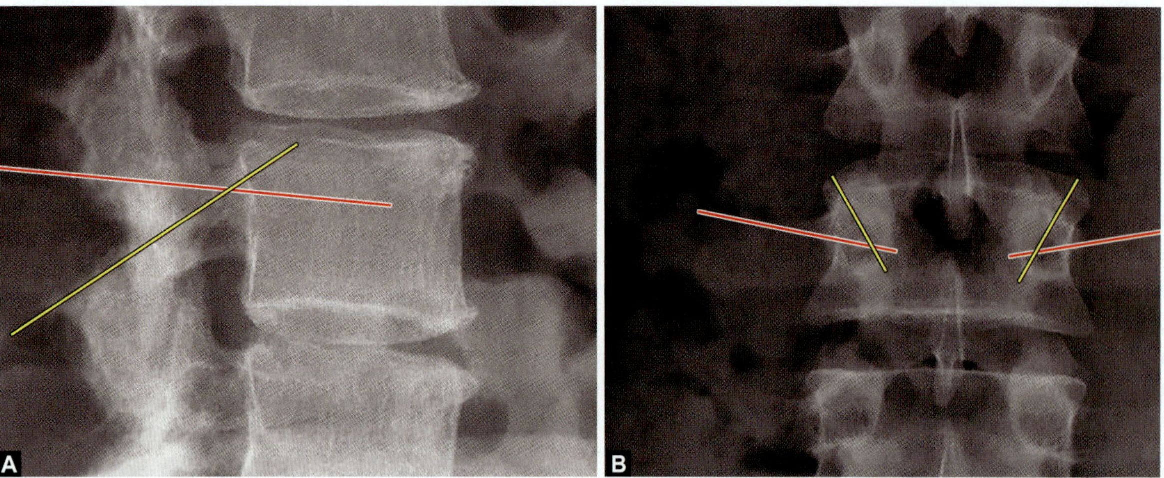

Figs. 10.2A and B: (A) A lateral lumbar radiograph demonstrating the desired caudad to cephalad trajectory for cortical screw placement (yellow) compared to traditional pedicle screw trajectory (red). (B) An anterior-posterior lumbar radiograph demonstrating the desired medial to lateral trajectory for cortical screw placement (yellow) compared to traditional pedicle screw trajectory (red).

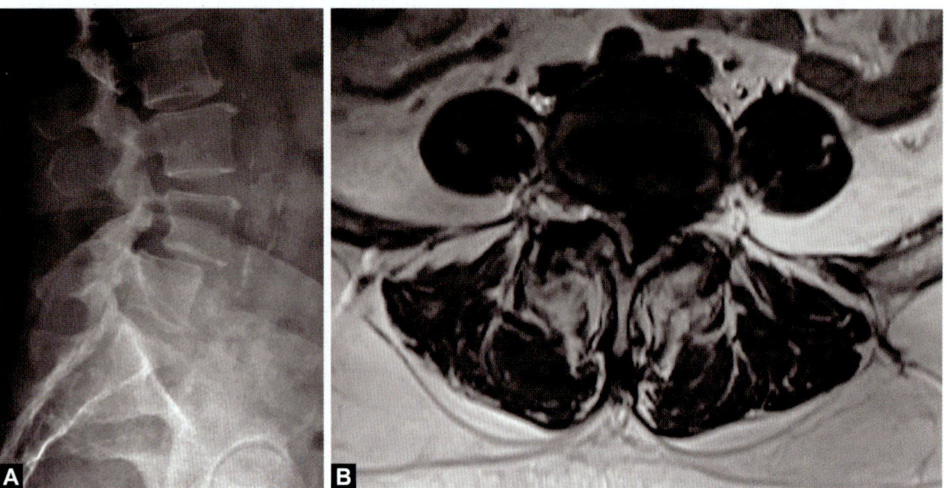

Figs. 10.3A and B: (A) A lateral lumbar radiograph demonstrating moderate multilevel degenerative changes with grade II spondylolisthesis at L4/5. (B) A T1-weighted axial MRI image at L4/5 level demonstrating moderate-to-severe tricompartmental stenosis.

in trauma settings. Cortical screws are a novel posterior instrumentation technique with benefits in patients with poor bone quality, MIS procedures, and demonstrate lower rates of facet violation potentially reducing the rate of adjacent segment disease.

CASE PRESENTATION

A 63-year-old female presents with several months of worsening lower back pain and bilateral leg radicular symptoms in the L5 nerve distribution. A physical examination demonstrates weakness in the left leg tibialis anterior and extensor hallucis longus with reduced sensation in the L5 distribution bilaterally. The MRI findings demonstrate grade two L4/5 degenerative spondylolisthesis with severe tricompartmental stenosis (Figs. 10.3A and B). The patients' symptoms have been refractory to nonoperative management including epidural steroid injections. She is indicated for a minimally invasive TLIF at the fourth and fifth lumbar vertebrae (Figs. 10.4 and 10.5).

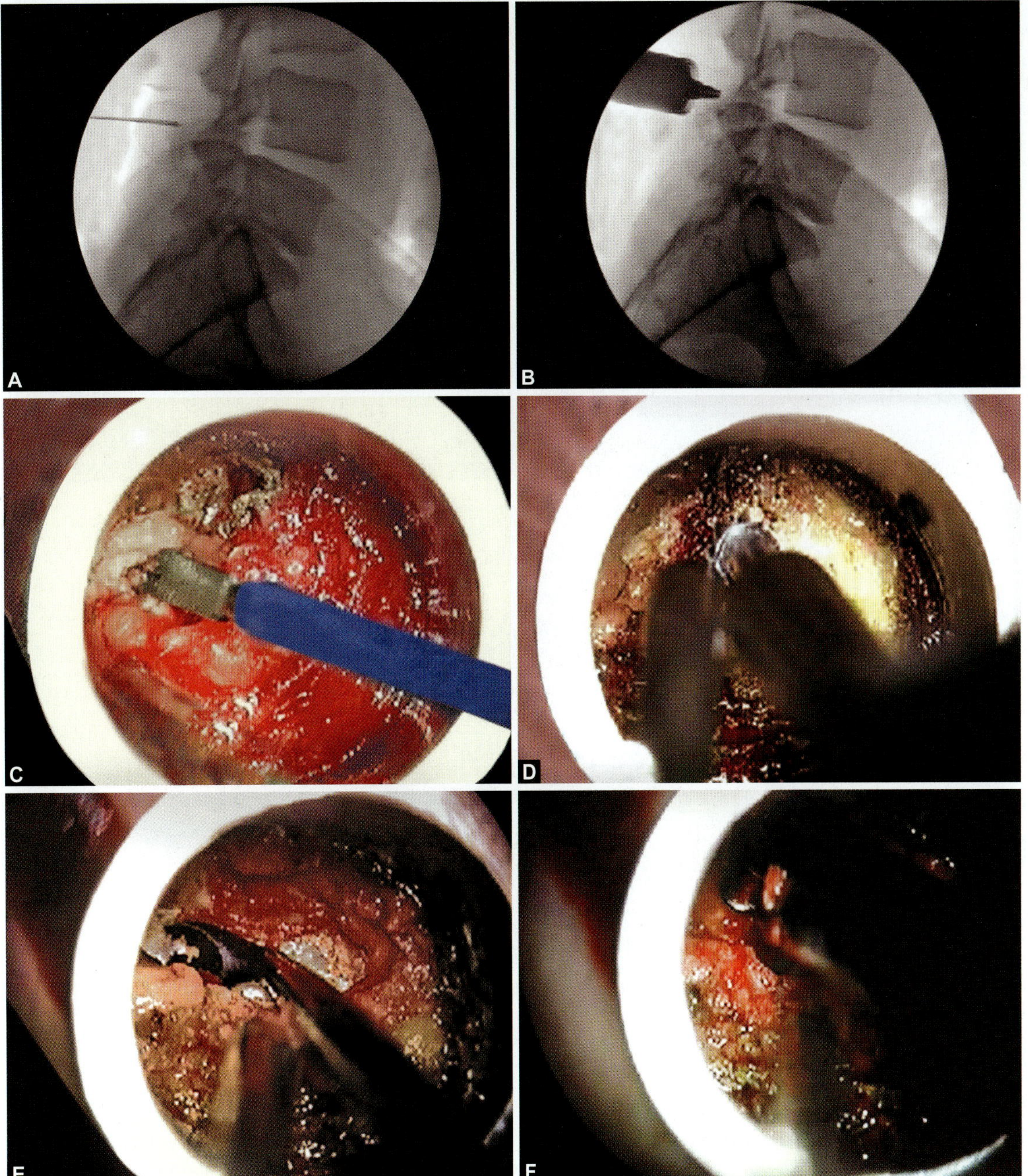

Figs. 10.4A to F: Following needle localization of the targeted disc space, a serial dilation is performed and the tube is docked in line (A and B). Following tube docking, subperiosteal dissection of the lamina and facet is performed with electrocautery (C). A high-speed burr is utilized to perform a laminectomy and expose ligamentum flavum (D). Ligamentum flavum is resected and a facetectomy is performed to gain access to the disc space (E and F).

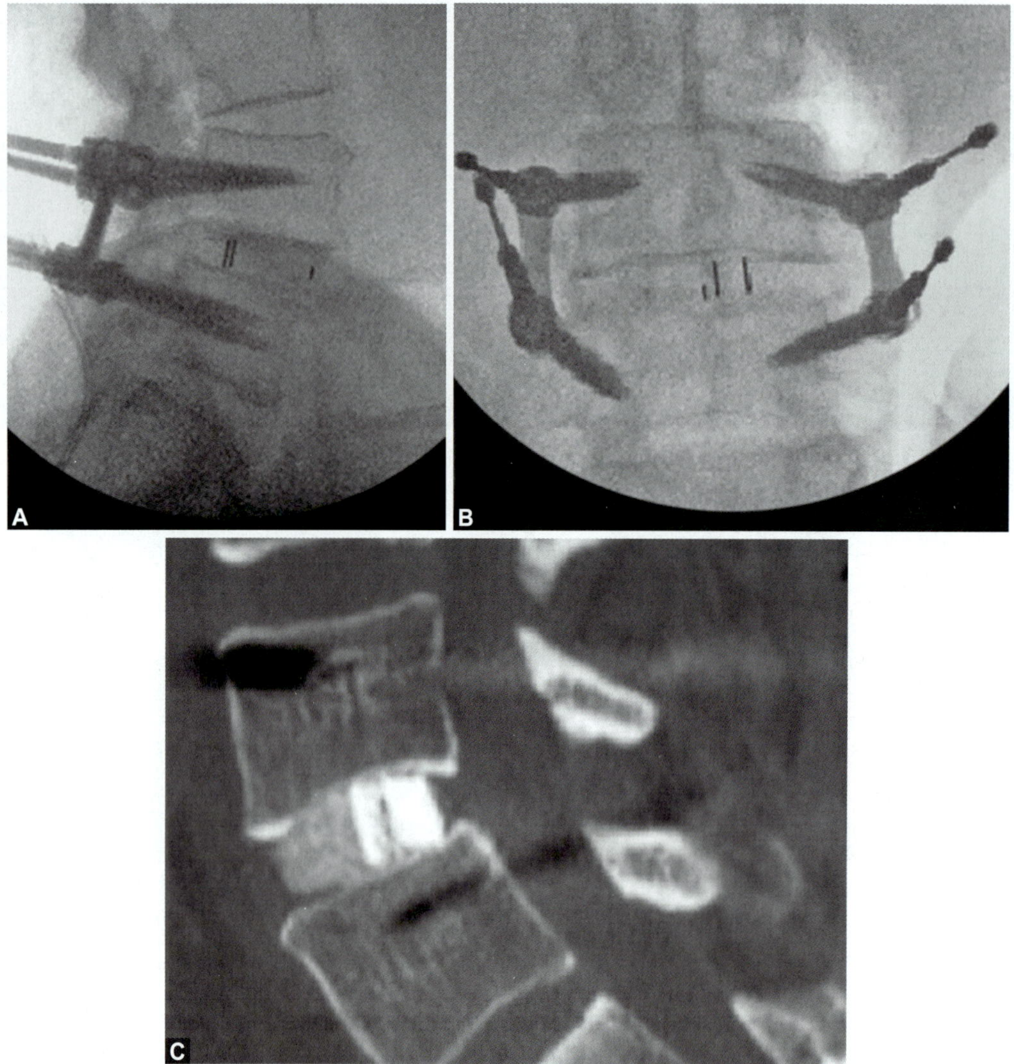

Figs. 10.5A to C: A careful disc preparation is the key to achieving fusion with minimally invasive surgical (MIS) transforaminal lumbar interbody fusion (TLIF). Dense packing of the disc space with allograft and appropriately sized and positioned TLIF cages is possible through MIS approaches (A and B). A follow-up CT scan at 3 months demonstrates solid fusion with an MIS TLIF technique (C).

REFERENCES

1. McAfee PC, Phillips FM, Andersson G, et al. Minimally invasive spine surgery. Spine. 2010;35(26 Suppl):S271-3.
2. Phillips FM, Cheng I, Rampersaud YR, et al. Breaking through the "glass ceiling" minimally invasive spine surgery. Spine. 2016;41 (Suppl 8):S39-43.
3. Kim CW. Scientific basis of minimally invasive spine surgery: Prevention of multifidus muscle injury during posterior lumbar surgery. Spine. 2010;35(26 Suppl):S281-6.
4. Peng CWB, Yue WM, Poh SY, et al. Clinical and radiological outcomes of minimally invasive versus open transforaminal lumbar interbody fusion. Spine. 2009;34(13):1385-9.

5. Lee KH, Yue WM, Yeo W, et al. Clinical and radiological outcomes of open versus minimally invasive transforaminal lumbar interbody fusion. Eur Spine J Off Publ Eur Spine Soc Eur Spinal Deform Soc Eur Sect Cerv Spine Res Soc. 2012;21(11):2265-70.
6. Seng C, Siddiqui MA, Wong KPL, et al. Five-year outcomes of minimally invasive versus open transforaminal lumbar interbody fusion: a matched-pair comparison study. Spine. 2013;38(23):2049-55. doi:10.1097/BRS.0b013e3182a8212d.
7. Goldstein CL, Phillips FM, Rampersaud YR. Comparative effectiveness and economic evaluations of open versus minimally invasive posterior or transforaminal lumbar interbody fusion: a systematic review. Spine. 2016;41(Suppl 8):S74-89.
8. Phan K, Rao PJ, Kam AC, et al. Minimally invasive versus open transforaminal lumbar interbody fusion for treatment of degenerative lumbar disease: Systematic review and meta-analysis. Eur Spine J Off Publ Eur Spine Soc Eur Spinal Deform Soc Eur Sect Cerv Spine Res Soc. 2015;24(5):1017-30.
9. Singh K, Nandyala SV, Marquez-Lara A, et al. A perioperative cost analysis comparing single-level minimally invasive and open transforaminal lumbar interbody fusion. Spine J Off J North Am Spine Soc. 2014;14(8):1694-701.
10. Nowitzke AM. Assessment of the learning curve for lumbar microendoscopic discectomy. Neurosurg. 2005;56(4):755-62.
11. Sclafani JA, Kim CW. Complications associated with the initial learning curve of minimally invasive spine surgery: a systematic review. Clin Orthop. 2014;472(6):1711-7.
12. Kim CW, Siemionow K, Anderson DG, et al. The current state of minimally invasive spine surgery. J Bone Jt Surg. 2011;93(6):353-70.
13. Nandyala SV, Fineberg SJ, Pelton M, et al. Minimally invasive transforaminal lumbar interbody fusion: One surgeon interbody fusion: Spine J. 2014;14(8):1460-5.
14. Lee JC, Jang H-D, Shin B-J. Learning curve and clinical outcomes of minimally invasive transforaminal lumbar interbody fusion: our experience in 86 consecutive cases. Spine. 2012;37(18):1548-57.
15. Park Y, Lee SB, Seok SO, et al. Perioperative surgical complications and learning curve associated with minimally invasive transforaminal lumbar interbody fusion: a single-institute experience. Clin Orthop Surg. 2015;7(1):91-6.
16. Kim CW, Lee Y-P, Taylor W, et al. Use of navigation-assisted fluoroscopy to decrease radiation exposure during minimally invasive spine surgery. Spine J Off J North Am Spine Soc. 2008;8(4):584-90.
17. Santoni BG, Hynes RA, McGilvray KC, et al. Cortical bone trajectory for lumbar pedicle screws. Spine J Off J North Am Spine Soc. 2009;9(5):366-73.
18. Davne SH, Myers DL. Complications of lumbar spinal fusion with transpedicular instrumentation. Spine. 1992;17(6 Suppl):S184-9.
19. Okuyama K, Sato K, Abe E, et al. Stability of transpedicle screwing for the osteoporotic spine. An in vitro study of the mechanical stability. Spine. 1993;18(15):2240-5.
20. Hirano T, Hasegawa K, Takahashi HE, et al. Structural characteristics of the pedicle and its role in screw stability. Spine. 1997;22(21):2504-9; discussion 2510.
21. Matsukawa K, Yato Y, Kato T, et al. In vivo analysis of insertional torque during pedicle screwing using cortical bone trajectory technique. Spine. 2014;39(4):E240-5.
22. Matsukawa K, Taguchi E, Yato Y, et al. Evaluation of the fixation strength of pedicle screws using cortical bone trajectory: what is the ideal trajectory for optimal fixation? Spine. 2015;40(15):E873-8.
23. Baluch DA, Patel AA, Lullo B, et al. Effect of physiological loads on cortical and traditional pedicle screw fixation. Spine. 2014;39(22):E1297-302.
24. Matsukawa K, Kato T, Yato Y, et al. Incidence and risk factors of adjacent cranial facet joint violation following pedicle screw insertion using cortical bone trajectory technique. Spine. 2016;41(14):E851-6.
25. Cardoso MJ, Dmitriev AE, Helgeson M, et al. Does superior-segment facet violation or laminectomy destabilize the adjacent level in lumbar transpedicular fixation? An in vitro human cadaveric assessment. Spine. 2008;33(26):2868-73.
26. Park P, Garton HJ, Gala VC, et al. Adjacent segment disease after lumbar or lumbosacral fusion: review of the literature. Spine. 2004;29(17):1938-44.
27. Sakaura H, Miwa T, Yamashita T, et al. Posterior lumbar interbody fusion with cortical bone trajectory screw fixation versus posterior lumbar interbody fusion using traditional pedicle screw fixation for degenerative lumbar spondylolisthesis: a comparative study. J Neurosurg Spine. 2016;25(5):591-5.

CHAPTER

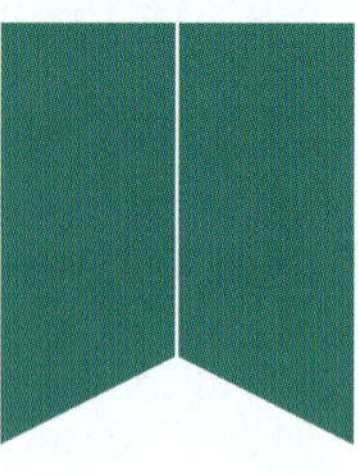

11

Lateral Lumbar Interbody Fusion

Mohammed Ali Alvi, Dennis P Kurian, Panagiotis Kerezoudis, Mohamad Bydon

INTRODUCTION

In recent years, minimally invasive spine (MIS) surgery has growing in popularity among both patients and surgeons. Specialized instruments and imaging modalities have allowed access to the spine without large incisions or extensive dissection. MIS approaches offer several advantages including less operative blood loss and tissue damage, shorter hospital stay and recovery time, and less postoperative pain over traditional open surgery. New MIS techniques have quickly emerged over the last decade for a wide range of spine conditions, but their growth has been somewhat impaired by surgical challenges. These include the steep learning curve associated with using endoscopic and percutaneous instruments, and the need for an access surgeon.[1]

Traditionally, common pathologic conditions of the lumbar spine are surgically treated by three distinct open approaches—(1) anterior lumbar interbody fusion (ALIF),[2-6] posterior lumbar interbody fusion (PLIF),[7] and transforaminal interbody fusion (TLIF).[8-11] A chosen approach determines patient positioning, relevant anatomy, and trajectory of instruments entering the disc space. The posterior approach involves accessing the disc space either medial to the facet joint or via the intervertebral foraminal space, allowing adequate visualization of nerve roots. Disadvantages include difficulty with endplate preparation, difficulty correcting coronal and sagittal balance, and risk of injury to posterior spinal nerves and musculature. The anterior approach requires an access surgeon to traverse the retroperitoneal space to expose the entire ventral surface for disc preparation. This approach carries an increased risk to vascular and visceral structures.[12]

Over the past decade, many alternative techniques have been introduced in the US with the aim to minimize surgical risks, decrease hospital length of stay and postoperative morbidity, and improve patient satisfaction.[6] One alternative technique is to approach the anterior lumbar spine laterally via a retroperitoneal access. In 1997, Micheal Mayer described a minimally invasive access to the disc space through a window between the peritoneum and psoas muscle. This technique is referred to as anterior-to-psoas (ATP) lateral interbody fusion. In 2006, Ozgur described another lateral technique to access the anterior lumbar spine through a transpsoas (TP) approach. An initial description of this technique was also presented by Pimenta in 2001.[13] Both these approaches have shown acceptable success in terms of patient outcomes and fusion rates while reducing approach related complications associated with anterior and posterior approaches. Both approaches have been increasingly employed in recent years as an effective option for degenerative conditions and deformities of the lumbar spine.

ANATOMY

The anterior lumbar spine is laterally accessed in the TP approach by dissecting through the psoas major muscle from a flank incision. Although dissection of the psoas is relatively straightforward, the lumbar plexus and major vessels are in close proximity to the surgical pathway. A preoperative magnetic resonance imaging

(MRI) can be used to delineate a surgical corridor by assessing the relation of neurovascular structures to the lower vertebral endplate.[14] A safe working zone for performing discectomy narrows from the L1-L2 interbody disc level to the L4-L5 level, with increasing sagittal overlap of structures meaning higher risk of neurologic and vascular injury at more caudal levels. In a normally aligned spine, the lumbar plexus migrates ventrally from the posterior of the vertebral body in relation to the sagittal lumbar spine as it moves caudally. Retroperitoneal blood vessels migrate dorsally and laterally from the anterior vertebral body as they move caudally.[15] Neurovasculature structures are generally in a safe distance from the radiographic center of the disc, but care must be taken to identify structural variants.[16] ATP, a more recent approach, accesses the lumbar spine between the peritoneum and the psoas muscle, avoiding both structures.[17]

The major innovation related to the ATP approach is accessing the Kambin's triangle through a minimally invasive access via a retroperitoneal path. The Kambin's triangle consists of the exiting nerve, superior border of the lower vertebra and the nerve root plus superior articular process.[18,19] The triangle is an electrophysiologically silent window, which allows the surgeon to access the lumbar spine without direct visualization.[20]

INDICATIONS

The TP approach efficiently provides deformity correction, comprehensive disc clearance, and decompression of foraminal stenosis.[12,21] It is a suitable option for degenerative conditions from the T12-L1 to L4-L5 vertebral body level. TP however, unlike ATP, cannot be used at the L5-S1 level due to anatomical obstruction of surgical access by the iliac crest and increased risk of injury by more laterally coursing iliac vessels and anteriorly coursing lumbar plexus nerves.[12,21] TP is a good option for deformity correction at the T12-L1 and L1-2 level, an excellent option at L2-3 and L3-4, and reasonable option at L4-5 but carries an increased risk of lumbar plexus or psoas injury. For degenerative spondylolisthesis, TP is associated with less complications, lower blood loss, and better restoration of disc height, segmental lumbar lordosis, and foraminal height.[12,22] TP has been shown to be an efficient technique for indirect decompression of foraminal stenosis with results equivalent to anterior and posterior interbody approaches. However, data for decompression of central canal and lateral stenosis are inconsistent.[21] TP is relatively contraindicated for patients with severe central canal stenosis, bony lateral recess stenosis, retroperitoneal abscesses or scarring, abnormal vascular anatomy, a low-lying L4-5 disc, severe osteoporosis, pregnancy, and active infection.[12,22]

Anterior-to-psoas is similarly indicated at the T12-L1 to L4-L5 level, but also is a suitable option at the L5-S1 level as it does not carry the same iatrogenic risk as TP. Indications for ATP include all degenerative indications and is also an excellent option for sagittal and coronal deformity correction especially in lumbar degenerative scoliosis with rotatory subluxations. The approach is contraindicated in patients with severe central canal stenosis and high-grade spondylolisthesis.[12] ATP has also been employed in cases where a previous fusion surgery resulting in pseudarthrosis or failure of fusion. For multilevel procedures, both approaches have been used but may require supplemental posterior osteotomies and pedicle screw/rod instrumentation.[12,22] The approach is now considered superior to posterior approaches for deformity cases with regard to magnitude of sagittal and coronal correction, disc height restoration, and indirect decompression of central and foraminal stenosis.[12,22] Other indications reported in the literature include thoracolumbar degenerative spondylolisthesis, lumbar degenerative disc disease, spinal stenosis, adjacent segment disease, pseudarthrosis, total disc arthroplasty conversion, anterior lumbar corpectomy, and revision of failed posterior procedures.[21,22]

TECHNIQUES

Transpsoas Approach

Patient Position and Preparation

The ideal position for the approach is a 90° right lateral decubitus position. For better access in upper lumbar levels, particularly it is recommended to flex the table or the patient, which creates some distance between the rib cage and iliac crest.[23] A mark is placed on the lateral side of the patient on a point overlying the center of the index disc-space. The anterior and posterior borders of the vertebral body are also marked.

Incision and Dissection

An oblique incision is made starting from the anterior and inferior end of the lower vertebral body extending posteriorly and superiorly toward the rostral vertebral body.[24] Blunt dissection of the subcutaneous tissue layer is made exposing the fibers of the external oblique muscle. The next layer is the internal oblique muscle whose fibers run in an opposite direction. These layers are split along the fibers to minimize injury to the abdominal nerves. The ilioinguinal and the iliohypogastric nerves which are located between the internal oblique and transverse abdominis are also protected.[25] Once the internal oblique layer is split, the transversalis fascia is visualized. Next, the retroperitoneal space is accessed by steady displacement of the peritoneum from posterior to anterior exposing the retroperitoneal fat and psoas muscle. A transpsoatic dissection uses continuous neuromonitoring to avoid any injury to the lumbar plexus which is in the substance of the psoas muscle. A K-wire, supplemented with the use of fluoroscopy helps to identify the correct lumbar level. Following this, specialized retractors designed for TP approaches are docked on the targeted disc space and are secured either by a table mounted articulating arm or vertebral fixation pins.

Discectomy and Cage Placement

Next, discectomy is performed using a combination of pituitary rongeurs, curettes, and paddle shavers. A Cobb elevator is passed along both endplates to the contralateral side avoiding any violation of the endplates.[25] Preparation of the entire surface of the endplate all the way across to the contralateral side is recommended because releasing the contralateral annulus improves exposure and allows for correction of coronal plane deformities.[24] Next, an intervertebral cage is gradually impacted into the bone and the position is verified on fluoroscopy. In order to prevent the risk of cage subsidence, it is recommended that the cage spans the entire width of the vertebral body resting on the ring apophysis and that overstuffing of the implant is avoided. The implant can either be left as a stand-alone device or supplemented with posterior instrumentation.

Anterior to Psoas Approach

Patient Positioning

Positioning and taping is identical to that for a TP approach. The patient is placed in lateral decubitus position. To relax the psoas muscle and femoral nerve, the hip is slightly flexed and positioned below the table break. A pillow can be placed in between the knees and lower pelvis, and tape is placed horizontally to the operating table over the greater trochanter and thigh to stabilize the positioning.[26] The skin is marked for incision above the level of pathology. It is recommended that the approach is left sided so that there is no need for venous traction.

Incision and Dissection

In left-sided ATP cases, the surgical window used for access approaches the disc space through the space between the common iliac vessels and psoas muscle. The skin incision is recommended to be centered on the disc space in the anterior one-third of the disc. Any incision on the skin should extend obliquely in the line with the external oblique muscle fibers.[26] This approximates to about 30 mm in front of the anterior superior iliac spine toward the umbilicus at L4-L5. Next, blunt dissection of the subcutaneous tissue is performed following which the external oblique fascia is cut in line exposing the abdominal muscle layer underneath.[26] The muscle layer is dissected in the line of their fibers taking care to avoid injuries to iliohypogastric and ilioinguinal nerves. Next, the transversalis fascia is opened laterally exposing the retroperitoneal fat. The fat is displaced backward using a pair of swabs on sticks. Once the retroperitoneal space is accessed, sequential dilators are introduced and docked into the disc-space anterior to psoas muscle and an access portal is established. The disc level is identified using a K-wire and fluoroscopy.

Discectomy and Cage Placement

Next, discectomy is performed using a drill and then shavers, ring curettes, long pituitary punches, and rasps all delivered through the access portal. Serial dilation of the rotating shavers helps with preparing the endplates. Violation of the endplates should be avoided as best as possible.[20] Then, trials of spacers are conducted to identify the right size and the cage is then impacted until one-third of it is past the midline, the cage is then rotated and further impacted into place until it is well centered on the AP and lateral fluoroscopic views. The choice of cage and supplementation with posterior instrumentation is as per the surgeon's preference.

OUTCOMES

Both approaches have been shown to have favorable clinical and radiographic outcomes. The TP approach is reported to have high fusion rates ranging from 88% to 98%.[23-25] The overall rate of postoperative transient neurologic events range from 0.6% to 33.6%.[4,26] The approach is reported to have better outcomes when supplemented with posterior fusion; stand-alone fusion using the approach has been reported to have less successful fusion rates. Marchi et al. and Watkins found a fusion rate of 86.5% and 73%, respectively with stand-alone TP fusion.[27,28] The cage size has also been shown to have an impact on outcomes. The wider cage size employed in TP approach compared to PLIF and TLIF is hypothesized to lead to improved spinal stability, better bone graft incorporation, and ultimately higher fusion rates.[25]

The TP approach has also been shown to be associated with significant improvement in patient reported outcomes. Alimi et al. demonstrated significant improvement in Oswestry disability index (ODI) and visual analog score (VAS) scores for back pain, buttock pain and leg pain postoperative and at last follow-up for patients with degenerative disc disease, spondylolisthesis, and degenerative scoliosis.[29] Castiavelli presented the results of 44 patients with single or multilevel degenerative lumbar stenosis showing 24%, 31%, and 67% change in right foraminal area, left foraminal area, and disc height, respectively. The authors also reported almost 50% and 40% improvement in VAS and ODI scores, respectively.[30] Lee et al. reported significant improvement in ODI and VAS scores in patients with spinal stenosis, spondylolisthesis and degenerative scoliosis. Tohmeh et al. found a 92% patient satisfaction rate in patients after a TP approach. Isaacs and Sombrano et al. presented the result of the only randomized trial where they compared TP fusion with TLIF.[31,32] They demonstrated generally favorable results with VAS back improvement of 73%, VAS leg improvement of 79%, and ODI improvement of 53%, which were all superior to the TLIF group.

The ATP approach has also shown generally positive outcomes. Mayer, who described the technique, reported favorable fusion rates, complication rates as well as operative factors such as total time and blood loss.[33] The approach has been compared to other techniques in observational studies. Kaiser et al. in 2002 compared outcomes with ATP to laparoscopic ALIF and found shorter operative length but more blood loss.[34] The approach was also compared to open ALIF by Saraph et al. in 2004 who found shorter operative time and less blood loss with ATP.[35] ATP has also been associated with positive patient reported outcomes. Ohtori et al. in 2015 presented a series of 12 patients with degenerative kyphoscoliosis and reported an improvement of 72% in VAS back pain and a 50% improvement in ODI score. The fusion rate was found to be 90% with none of the patients requiring revision surgery.[36] Lin et al. presented their analysis of 46 patients with disc herniation, spondylolisthesis, and pseudarthrosis and found a fusion rate of 94.2%; improvement in VAS and Roland-Morris questionnaire scores by 68% and 55%; and a satisfaction rate of 87%.[37]

COMPLICATIONS

The most common complications of TP are neurologic in nature, including anterior thigh pain or weakness and psoas mechanical deficit.[22] These transient plexopathies may occur from iatrogenic injury to the psoas muscle or neuropraxia. However, these deficits persist in a much smaller percentage of patients. Whereas 28.7% of patients have sensory deficits and 41% have anterior thigh/groin pain 6 weeks after surgery, only 1.6% and 0.8% have sensory deficits and pain respectively after 12 months.[16] Similarly, Kwon et al. found that patients in the immediate postoperative period reported a 38% incidence of sensory deficit and a 24% incidence of extremity weakness, which decreased to 9.6% and 3.2%, respectively at a minimum of 18 months follow-up. Higher rates of early neurologic complications were observed with surgery at the L4/5 level, but were not significant at 18 months follow-up.[38] Risk varies depending on the approached levels and operative time, with multilevel fusions and prolonged duration of surgery carrying increased risk of neurologic complication.[16] ATP carries a much lower risk of psoas and lumbar plexus injury since the psoas is not surgically dissected.[12]

As retroperitoneal approaches, TP and ATP pose increased risk for the vascular and visceral structures coursing. Serious vascular and wound risks include psoas hematoma, venous laceration, arterial thrombosis, and pseudoaneurysm.[12,39] Visceral complications such as bowel perforation occur at a rate of 0.16–0.83% and ureter injury at a rate of 0.1–0.8%.[39,40]

Nonneurologic complications are notable using the lateral approach. The three most predominant are pseudarthrosis, subsidence, and fractures. The rate of pseudarthrosis is reported at 5% and cage subsidence at 7% in the literature.[39] Kwon et al. reported a subsidence rate of 14%, with higher rates associated with the narrower 18 mm cage compared to the 22 mm cage.[41-44] Additional rare complications include abdominal wall asymmetry, urinary retention, and atrial fibrillation.[22]

CASE PRESENTATION

Case 1

History

A 59-year-old female presenting with a 5-year history of mild, intermittent lower back pain aggravated by walking and prolonged standing, relieved by bending forward and rest. 3 months prior to presentation her symptoms started to significantly worsen. Radiographs revealed a grade 1 anterolisthesis of L4 on L5 and instability on flexion-extension (Fig. 11.1A). MRI showed evidence of stenosis at the L4 interspace secondary to advanced spondylosis, along with bilateral degenerative neural foraminal narrowing (Fig. 11.1B). Due to her symptomatic progression as well as the findings of instability and severe stenosis, it was opted to proceed with surgical intervention.

Operative Course

Under general anesthesia, the patient was placed in a lateral position with the left side up. All pressure points were padded and the patient was prepped and draped in a sterile fashion. An O-arm spin was performed to confirm localization. A left-sided lateral incision was made followed by dissection to expose the external oblique, internal oblique, and transversalis muscle. After the transversalis fascia was dissected, the retroperitoneal space was accessed and sequential dilators were utilized to facilitate the approach. Finally, the psoas muscle was identified and the tubes were advanced *anterior* to it down to the L4-L5 disc space. Upon arriving at the disc space, a K-wire was entered into the disc and fluoroscopic images were taken to confirm the level. Next, an L4 discectomy was performed and a 12° lordotic, 12 mm × 45 mm × 20 mm cage was placed which was filled with 6 cc of bone matrix. Next, a large plate and two 5.5 mm × 35 mm screws were placed, one at the level of L4 and the other at L5. Free-run electromyography (EMG) from bilateral L3-S1 muscles was monitored intraoperatively with no concerning signs (Figs. 11.1C and D).

Postoperative Course

The patient had an uneventful postoperative recovery period and was able to ambulate the same day and discharged on postoperative day 1. On follow-up at 6 weeks, she was off all pain medication with her leg symptoms resolved and normal activity restored. X-rays revealed instrumentation in a good position without evidence of loosening or failure (Fig. 11.1E). On subsequent follow-up at 12 weeks and 6 months, she continued to do well, had complete symptomatic resolution and imaging revealed instrumentation in place with no evidence of loosening or failure and improvement of the anterolisthesis.

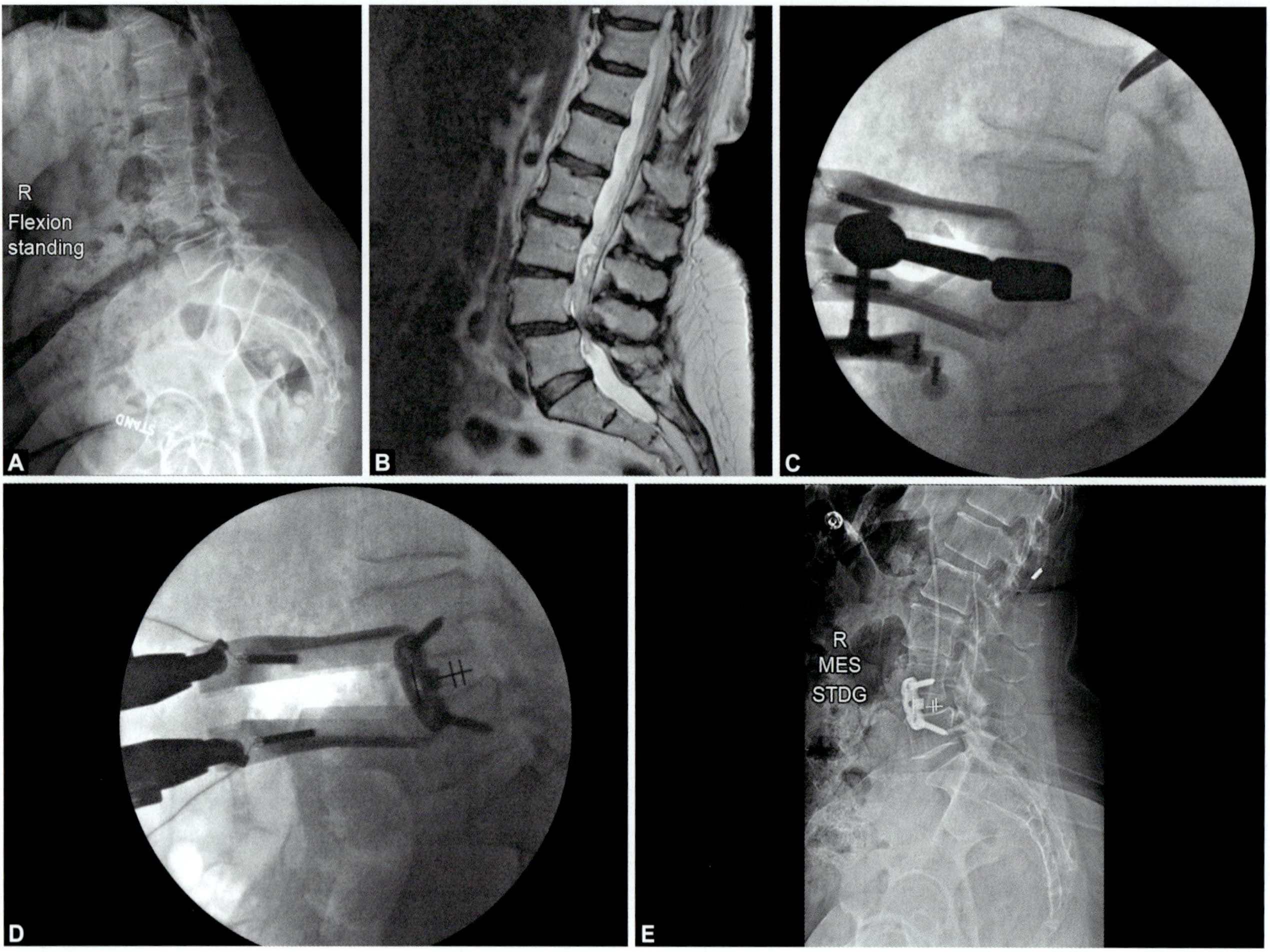

Figs. 11.1A to E: (A) Preoperative lateral extension X-ray showing grade 1 anterolisthesis of L4 on L5; (B) preoperative MRI showing evidence of severe central canal stenosis with cauda equina compression at the L4 interspace secondary to advanced spondylosis, along with bilateral degenerative neural foraminal narrowing; (C) intraoperative fluoroscopy showing portal with instruments in the disc space; (D) intraoperative fluoroscopy showing placement of cage; (E) postoperative lateral X-ray.

Case 2

History

A 61-year-old male with a history of L4-L5 laminectomy and fusion of L4-5 3 years ago presented with persistent lower back pain, radiculopathy signs including numbness and pain in the legs bilaterally, as well as neurogenic claudication. The symptoms were suggestive of postlaminectomy syndrome or adjacent segment stenosis at L3-L4. An EMG was performed which showed L5-S1 radiculopathies bilaterally. An MRI revealed adjacent segment disease at L3-L4 (Figs. 11.2A and B).

Operative Course

The patient was intubated under general endotracheal anesthesia and was positioned lateral. A reference frame was placed and O-arm spin along with stereotactic navigation were used to mark the L3 and L4 vertebral bodies. An incision was made two fingerbreadths anterior to the mark. Dissection was continued through the external oblique fascia, the external oblique, internal oblique, and transversalis muscle. The retroperitoneal space was accessed and subsequently the prevertebral fascia was approached. The dissection was continued to enter the prepsoas space.

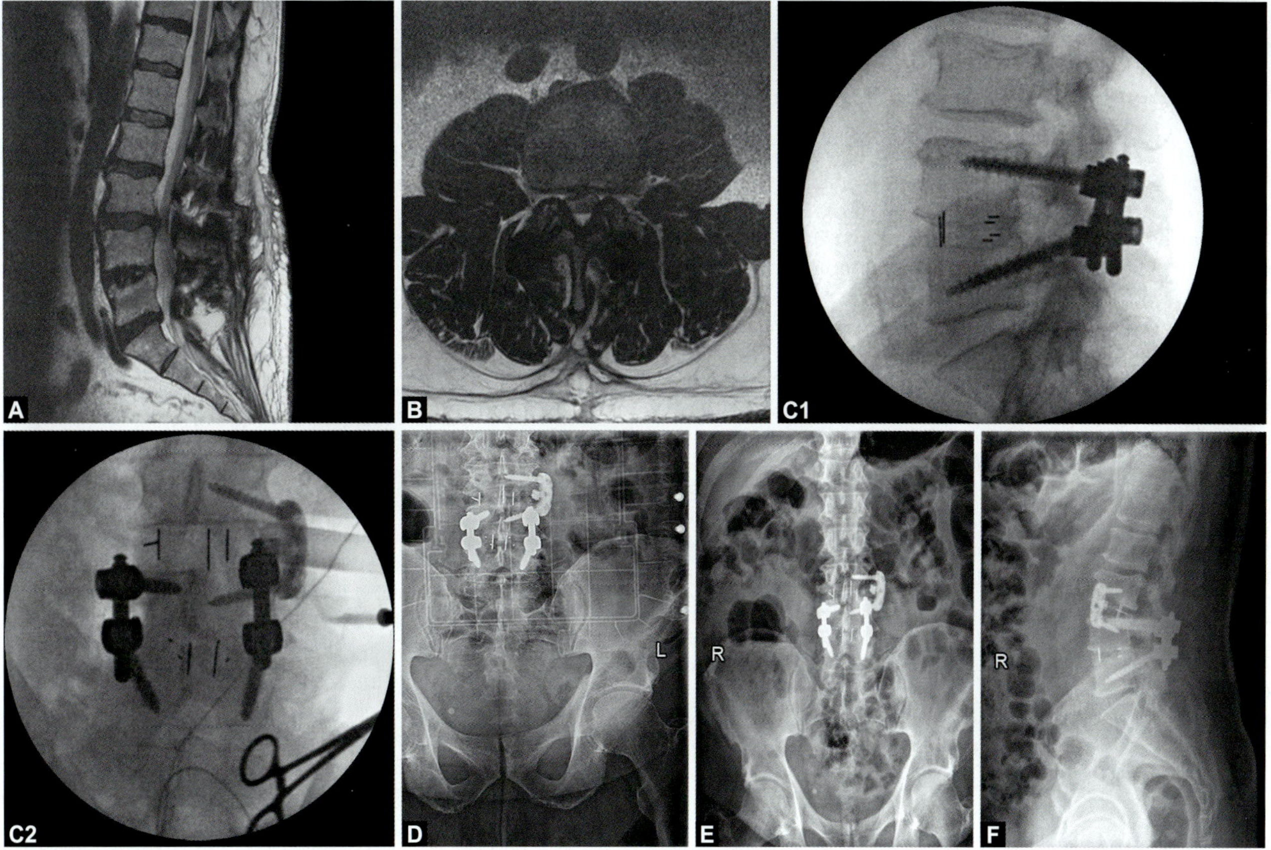

Figs. 11.2A to F: Preoperative MRI: (A) Sagittal and (B) axial showing adjacent segment disease at L3-L4; (C) intraoperative fluoroscopy showing placement of intervertebral cage and posterior instrumentation; (D) postoperative anteroposterior (AP) X-ray showing well-placed instrumentation; (E) AP and (F) lateral X-ray 3 months postoperative showing intact instrumentation.

At this point, sequential tubular dilators were placed along with light source. Next, a discectomy was performed at L3-4 using Cobb dilator which traversed through the disc space into the contralateral annulus thus removing a significant part of the disc. After adequate discectomy, the endplates were decorticated to prepare for arthrodesis. A minimally invasive ATP measuring 14 mm × 55 mm and 12° lordotic was placed at L3-L4 along two 35 mm screws, one at the L3 body and one at the L4 body (Fig. 11.2C). Inside the cage was placed cancellous chips as well as 1 cc of cellular bone matrix.

Postoperative Course

The patient had an uneventful postoperative course and was ambulating on postoperative day 1. His pain was well controlled and was subsequently discharged. Postoperative imaging revealed well-placed instrumentation without any loosening of screw or mal-positioned cage (Fig. 11.2D). Similarly, at 3 months follow-up, patient reported resolution of pain and imaging revealed well-positioned instrumentation (Figs. 11.2E and F).

REFERENCES

1. Ozgur BM, Aryan HE, Pimenta L, et al. Extreme lateral interbody fusion (XLIF): A novel surgical technique for anterior lumbar interbody fusion. Spine J. 2006;6:435-43.
2. Brau SA, Delamarter RB, Schiffman ML, et al. Vascular injury during anterior lumbar surgery. Spine J. 2004;4:409-12.
3. Fantini GA, Pappou IP, Girardi FP, et al. Major vascular injury during anterior lumbar spinal surgery: Incidence, risk factors, and management. Spine. 2007;32:2751-8.
4. Rodgers WB, Gerber EJ, Patterson J. Intraoperative and early postoperative complications in extreme lateral interbody fusion: an analysis of 600 cases. Spine. 2011;36:26-32.
5. Rajaraman V, Vingan R, Roth P, et al. Visceral and vascular complications resulting from anterior lumbar interbody fusion. J Neurosurg. 1999;91:60-4.

6. Sofianos DA, Briseño MR, Abrams J, et al. Complications of the lateral transpsoas approach for lumbar interbody arthrodesis: a case series and literature review. Clin Orthop Relat Res. 2012;470:1621-32.
7. DiPaola CP, Molinari RW. Posterior lumbar interbody fusion. J Am Acad Orthop Surg. 2008;16:130-9.
8. Dhall SS, Wang MY, Mummaneni PV. Clinical and radiographic comparison of mini-open transforaminal lumbar interbody fusion with open transforaminal lumbar interbody fusion in 42 patients with long-term follow-up. J Neurosurg Spine. 2008;9:560-5.
9. Park P, Foley KT. Minimally invasive transforaminal lumbar interbody fusion with reduction of spondylolisthesis: technique and outcomes after a minimum of 2 years' follow-up. Neurosurg Focus. 2008;25:E16.
10. Rihn JA, Patel R, Makda J, et al. Complications associated with single-level transforaminal lumbar interbody fusion. Spine J. 2009;9:623-9.
11. Villavicencio AT, Burneikiene S, Bulsara KR, et al. Perioperative complications in transforaminal lumbar interbody fusion versus anterior-posterior reconstruction for lumbar disc degeneration and instability. J Spinal Disord Tech. 2006;19:92-7.
12. Mobbs RJ, Phan K, Malham G, et al. Lumbar interbody fusion: techniques, indications and comparison of interbody fusion options including PLIF, TLIF, MI-TLIF, OLIF/ATP, LLIF and ALIF. J Spine Surg. 2015;1:2-18.
13. Pimenta L. Lateral endoscopic transpsoas retroperitoneal approach for spine surgery. Paper presented at VIII Brazilian Spine Society Meeting. Belo Horizonte, Minas Gerais, Brazil (2001).
14. Uribe JS, Arredondo N, Dakwar E, et al. Defining the safe working zones using the minimally invasive lateral retroperitoneal transpsoas approach: an anatomical study. J Neurosurg Spine. 2010;13:260-6.
15. Regev GJ, Chen L, Dhawan M, et al. Morphometric analysis of the ventral nerve roots and retroperitoneal vessels with respect to the minimally invasive lateral approach in normal and deformed spines. Spine. 2009;34:1330-5.
16. Pumberger M, Hughes AP, Huang RR, et al. Neurologic deficit following lateral lumbar interbody fusion. Eur Spine J. 2012;21:1192-9.
17. Phan K, Huo YR, Hogan JA, et al. Minimally invasive surgery in adult degenerative scoliosis: a systematic review and meta-analysis of decompression, anterior/lateral and posterior lumbar approaches. J Spine Surg. 2016;2:89-104.
18. Kambin P, Zhou L. Arthroscopic discectomy of the lumbar spine. Clin Orthop Relat Res. 1997;337:49-57.
19. Kambin P, Sampson S. Posterolateral percutaneous suction-excision of herniated lumbar intervertebral discs. Report of interim results. Clin Orthop Relat Res. 1986;207:37-43.
20. Abbasi H, Abbasi A. Oblique lateral lumbar interbody fusion (OLLIF): technical notes and early results of a single surgeon comparative study. Cureus. 2015;7:e351.
21. Lang G, Perrech M, Navarro-Ramirez R, et al. Potential and limitations of neural decompression in extreme lateral interbody fusion—a systematic review. World Neurosurg. 2017;101:99-113.
22. Pawar AY, Hughes AP, Sama AA, et al. A comparative study of lateral lumbar interbody fusion and posterior lumbar interbody fusion in degenerative lumbar spondylolisthesis. Asian Spine J. 2015;9:668-74.
23. Bentley G. European surgical orthopaedics and traumatology: The EFORT textbook. Berlin, Heidelberg: Springer; 2014.
24. Pawar A, Hughes A, Girardi F, et al. Lateral lumbar interbody fusion. Asian Spine J. 2015;9:978-83.
25. Singh K, Vaccaro AR. Pocket atlas of spine surgery. Thieme; 2012.
26. Gragnaniello C, Seex K. Anterior to psoas (ATP) fusion of the lumbar spine: evolution of a technique facilitated by changes in equipment. J Spine Surg. 2016;2:256-65.
27. Sharma AK, Kepler CK, Girardi FP, et al. Lateral lumbar interbody fusion: clinical and radiographic outcomes at 1 year: a preliminary report. J Spinal Disord Tech. 2011;24:242-50.
28. Dakwar E, Cardona RF, Smith DA, et al. Early outcomes and safety of the minimally invasive, lateral retroperitoneal transpsoas approach for adult degenerative scoliosis. Neurosurg Focus. 2010;28:E8.
29. Waddell B, Briski D, Qadir R, et al. Lateral lumbar interbody fusion for the correction of spondylolisthesis and adult degenerative scoliosis in high-risk patients: early radiographic results and complications. Ochsner J. 2014;14:23-31.
30. Youssef JA, McAfee PC, Patty CA, et al. Minimally invasive surgery: lateral approach interbody fusion: results and review. Spine. 2010;35:S302-11.
31. Watkins R 4th, Watkins R 3rd, Hanna R. Non-union rate with stand-alone lateral lumbar interbody fusion. Medicine. 2014;93:e275.
32. Marchi L, Abdala N, Oliveira L, et al. Stand-alone lateral interbody fusion for the treatment of low-grade degenerative spondylolisthesis. Scientific World J. 2012;2012:456346.
33. Alimi M, Hofstetter CP, Cong GT, et al. Radiological and clinical outcomes following extreme lateral interbody fusion. J Neurosurg Spine. 2014;20:623-35.
34. Castellvi AE, Nienke TW, Marulanda GA, et al. Indirect decompression of lumbar stenosis with transpsoas interbody cages and percutaneous posterior instrumentation. Clin Orthop Relat Res. 2014;472:1784-91.
35. Sembrano JN, Tohmeh A, Isaacs R, et al. Two-year comparative outcomes of MIS lateral and MIS transforaminal interbody fusion in the treatment of degenerative spondylolisthesis: Part I: Clinical findings. Spine. 2016;41(Suppl 8):S123-32.
36. Isaacs RE, Sembrano JN, Tohmeh AG, et al. Two-year comparative outcomes of MIS lateral and MIS transforaminal interbody fusion in the treatment of degenerative spondylolisthesis: Part II: Radiographic findings. Spine. 2016;41(Suppl 8):S133-44.
37. Mayer HM. A new microsurgical technique for minimally invasive anterior lumbar interbody fusion. Spine. 1997;22:691-9; discussion 700.
38. Kaiser MG, Haid RW Jr, Subach BR, et al. Comparison of the mini-open versus laparoscopic approach for anterior lumbar interbody fusion: a retrospective review. Neurosurg. 2002;51:97-103; discussion 103-5.
39. Saraph V, Lerch C, Walochnik N, et al. Comparison of conventional versus minimally invasive extraperitoneal approach for anterior lumbar interbody fusion. Eur Spine J. 2004;13:425-31.
40. Ohtori S, Orita S, Yamauchi K, et al. Mini-open anterior retroperitoneal lumbar interbody fusion: oblique lateral interbody fusion for degenerated lumbar spinal kyphoscoliosis. Asian Spine J. 2015;9:565-72.
41. Lin J-F, Iundusi R, Tarantino U, et al. Intravertebral plate and cage system via lateral trajectory for lumbar interbody fusion—a novel fixation device. Spine J. 2010;10:S86.
42. Kwon B, Kim DH. Lateral lumbar interbody fusion: indications, outcomes, and complications. J Am Acad Orthop Surg. 2016;24:96-105.
43. Hijji FY, Narain AS, Bohl DD, et al. Lateral lumbar interbody fusion: a systematic review of complication rates. Spine J. 2017;17(10):1412-9. doi:10.1016/j.spinee.2017.04.022.
44. Fujibayashi S, Kawakami N, Asazuma T, et al. Complications associated with lateral interbody fusion: nationwide survey of 2998 cases during the first two years of its use in Japan. Spine. 2017;42(19):1478-84.

CHAPTER

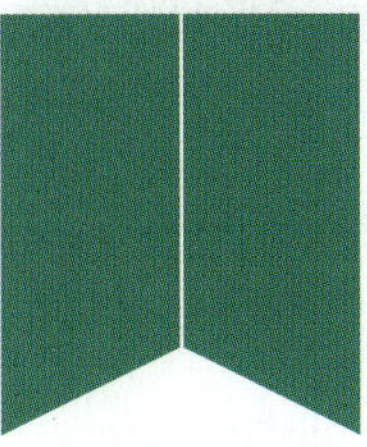

12

Pedicle Subtraction Osteotomy

Arjun Sebastian, Alexander R Vaccaro

INTRODUCTION

Adult sagittal deformity results from fixed sagittal imbalance that can occur from a loss of lumbar lordosis or progression of thoracic kyphosis. Initially described as a technique for the treatment of fixed sagittal deformity in ankylosing spondylitis,[1] the pedicle subtraction osteotomy (PSO) has become a popular technique to manage kyphotic deformities resulting from other etiologies. Using a single posterior approach, this powerful corrective osteotomy can achieve up to 35° of lordosis and 10 cm of posterior trunk translation.[2] Understanding the appropriate indications, preoperative planning, and potential pitfalls, associated with this technique, is critical to achieving a successful outcome with this complex procedure.

ETIOLOGY

Understanding normal sagittal alignment is critical to evaluating patients with fixed sagittal deformities. A wide range of lumbar lordosis has been described in asymptomatic individuals to be between 14° and 69°.[3] On average total lordosis is around 60° in asymptomatic individuals with slightly less lordosis in patients with mechanical back pain.[4] Overall, over 60% of total lumbar lordosis is achieved at the L4-5 and L5-S1 segments. Despite this, patients with a loss of lordosis are able to compensate with proximal lumbar hyperlordosis. Normal alignment in the sagittal plane requires the head to be balanced over the pelvis. This results in the gravity plumb line from the center of the C7 vertebral body falling at the posterior corner of the S1 endplate.[5,6]

There are several potential causes of fixed sagittal imbalance. Harrington rod constructs were popular three to four decades ago for the treatment of adolescent idiopathic scoliosis. For double major curves, traditional constructs started in the proximal thoracic spine and typically ended at L3 or L4. These Harrington constructs relied on intervertebral distraction for curvature correction. As a result, this resulted in proximal lumbar hypolordosis at the distal end of the construct. While patients initially were able to maintain normal sagittal alignment with compensation and hyperlordosis at the distal unfused segments, over time progressive disc degeneration and collapse from adjacent segment disease lead to a loss of lordosis and positive sagittal balance. This process occurs on average two to four decades after the index surgery.[7-9]

Sagittal imbalance can also occur in patients with post-traumatic deformities. Patients who sustain burst fractures or severe compression fractures especially in the thoracolumbar spine can develop a marked local kyphosis at the fracture site. These angular deformities can worsen over time as adjacent discs degenerate leading to collapse and worsening kyphosis.[8]

One of the original indications for osteotomy was for sagittal imbalance occurring in the setting of ankylosing spondylitis. This inflammatory spine condition results in an enthesopathy with progressive bony destruction at tendon insertion sites. This leads to pannus formation, new bone formation, and ankyloses resulting in marginal syndesmophyte formation and progressive fusion of disc spaces leading to loss of lumbar lordosis. The result is a stiff spinal deformity that patients are unable to compensate for.[1,7]

Lastly, another cause of fixed sagittal imbalance can result from the previous treatment of degenerative spinal conditions. Patients who underwent previous lumbar decompression may develop instability and progressive disc collapse with kyphosis. Similarly, patients who underwent previous lumbar fusion may also develop sagittal imbalance if fused in hypolordosis.[8]

EVALUATION

When evaluating patients with sagittal imbalance in addition to assessing potential etiology, it is critical to obtain a thorough history. Clinicians should differentiate back and lower extremity pain as well as determine issues with mobility, alignment, and forward gaze. Patients with sagittal imbalance report intractable back pain particularly with standing or walking and decreased functional capacity. A complete assessment of medical comorbidities including cardiopulmonary issues, diabetes, obesity, and osteoporosis should be performed so that patients may be optimized medically prior to any procedure. A complete surgical history should also be obtained with attention paid to previous decompressed and fused levels as well as any history of prior surgical site infections.[10-12]

On physical examination, it is important to assess standing alignment as well as gait. It is critical when assessing standing alignment that the knees are in a fully extended position. Patients with positive sagittal balance often compensate by retroversion of the pelvis, hip extension, and knee flexion to maintain forward gaze. These compensatory mechanisms lead to quadriceps fatigue and limited standing and walking tolerance. All of these factors lead to gait instability and progressive functional disability. In addition to standing alignment, it is critical to assess alignment in the supine position to determine any hip or knee contractures. It is also helpful to assess supine alignment to determine how fixed the kyphotic deformity is. Along with an assessment of alignment, all patients require a full neurologic evaluation. In particular, any signs of myelopathy such as a Hoffmann sign or hyperreflexia should be assessed further.[2,10]

Radiographic workup requires long standing X-rays in the anteroposterior (AP) and lateral planes. Proper assessment of alignment requires the knees to be fully extended and hands positioned on the ipsilateral clavicles. Flexion and extension X-rays should also be obtained to assess the flexibility of the deformity. If any coronal deformity is appreciated, side bending films may also be obtained. Several radiographic measures are critical for proper assessment of sagittal deformity and preoperative planning. The sagittal vertical axis (SVA) or C7 plumb line normally passes through the posterior aspect of the sacral endplate. Positive balance is considered when the C7 plumb line falls anterior to the L5-S1 disc space. SVA greater than 5 cm is considered abnormal and is associated with poorer health related quality of life outcomes.[5,6,13] Other important measurements include lumbar lordosis (Cobb angle of the inferior endplate of T12 to the superior endplate of S1), pelvic incidence (angle between the perpendicular to the sacral endplate and midpoint of the femoral heads), and pelvic tilt (angle between the midpoint of the sacral endplate, midpoint of the femoral heads, and the vertical axis) (Figs. 12.1A and B). Lumbopelvic mismatch assessed as a difference between pelvic incidence and lumbar lordosis is normally less than 10° but increases with hypolordosis. Similarly, pelvic tilt is normally less than 20° but increases with positive sagittal balance due to compensatory pelvic retroversion.[9,11,14,15]

Magnetic resonance imaging is helpful for the assessment of concurrent lumbar stenosis as well as evaluating the neural elements at the planned sites of osteotomy. Given that many patients with fixed deformities have undergone previous lumbar surgery, it is important to assess prior decompressions for dural morphology and epidural fibrosis. Computed tomography scans, while helpful for assessing pedicle morphology and extent of previous laminectomy sites, are not routinely required for preoperative assessment.[2]

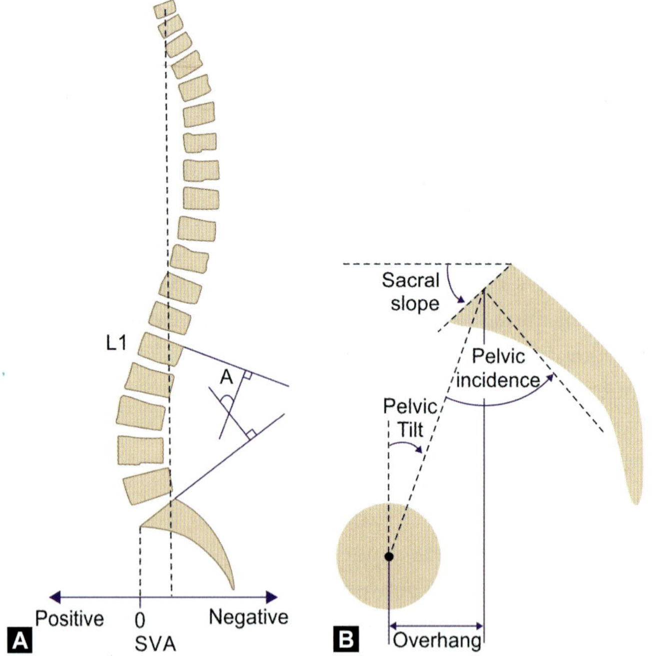

Figs. 12.1A and B: (A) C7 plumb line showing the sagittal vertical axis measurement and positive versus negative sagittal balance. The Cobb angle demonstrates the calculation of lumbar lordosis. (B) the measurement of pelvic parameters include pelvic tilt, pelvic incidence, and sacral slope (SVA: sagittal vertical axis).

Source: Joseph SA Jr, Moreno AP, Brandoff J, et al. Sagittal plane deformity in the adult patient. Journal of the American Academy of Orthopaedic Surgeons (JAAOS). 2009;17(6):378-88.

INDICATIONS

Patients with fixed sagittal imbalance rarely require surgical intervention. Patients should always undergo comprehensive nonoperative management first including nonsteroidal anti-inflammatory medications, physical therapy, and activity modification. If those conservative treatments fail, and the patient's symptoms are causing significant functional disability to limit activities of daily living, surgical management should be considered. Important considerations for surgical planning include assessment of the flexibility of the deformity, the focus of the kyphosis, and levels needing fusion with the goals being to minimize pseudarthrosis and junctional breakdown. Treatment options include multilevel interbody fusions, Smith-Petersen osteotomy (SPO), PSO, and vertebral column resection (VCR). Multilevel interbody fusions or SPOs are reserved for patients with multisegment rounded kyphosis. These techniques may be used in combination with each other and to supplement other osteotomy techniques. Critical to the success of SPO is the flexibility of the disc space as the osteotomy hinges on extension at the disc space to create lordosis. In contrast, PSO and VCR are reserved for fixed deformities typically with a sharper more angular kyphotic deformity. PSO may also be considered in patients with sweeping deformities that lack disc space mobility, such as patients with ankylosing spondylitis or previous fusion. PSO and VCR are generally utilized in patients with an SVA greater than 10 cm with VCR being typically utilized in the thoracic spine and PSO in the lumbar spine.[16,17]

Pedicle subtraction osteotomy results in correction of sagittal deformity entirely through one vertebral body and involves correction through all three columns. Tracing paper may be utilized for preoperative planning of the wedge resection. Surgeons can reliably expect to achieve 30° of lumbar lordosis and roughly 10 cm of sagittal translation.[2,18] While SPOs may be utilized to augment lordosis (at roughly 10° per level), for patients with deformities requiring more than 60° of correction, consideration should be given to a two-level PSO.[19] A single-level PSO is typically performed at L3 or L4. L3 PSO has the advantage of being central in the lumbar spine and providing additional distal fixation points, while L4 PSO provides lordotic correction distally which is more consistent with physiologic alignment.

TECHNIQUE

Following induction of anesthesia and intubation, the patient is positioned prone on a Jackson table. Care is taken to pad all bony prominences and leave the hips in slight flexion so that they may be extended to facilitate osteotomy closure. The authors prefer to use neuromonitoring with both somatosensory and motor evoked potentials. Following this, a routine dorsal exposure of the spine is performed. In the setting of previous decompression, care should be taken to avoid incidental durotomy. However, epidural scar tissue will need to be carefully resected in this situation to allow for adequate mobilization of the thecal sac to perform the osteotomy. A subperiosteal dissection of the facets and transverse processes should be performed.

Following exposure, pedicle screw placement should be performed. The authors recommend obtaining at least three points of fixation above and below the osteotomy site. Since junctional breakdown is common when ending fusions at the thoracolumbar junction, this often requires extending proximal fixation to T10 or T11. Distally, ending long constructs at S1 often result in distal junctional failure and thus the authors prefer to extend the fusion to the pelvis in the absence of a fused L5-S1 segment.[20-22]

When performing pelvic fixation, iliac bolts and S2-alar-ilium (S2AI) screws are both available as options. Iliac bolts are started in the posterior superior iliac spine and angulated laterally and caudally toward the greater trochanter. While achieving excellent fixation in the ilium, these screws typically require offset connectors and cause hardware prominence. As a result, the authors favor the S2AI technique. This technique requires exposure of the S1 and S2 foramen. The starting point for the screw is at the midpoint between the foramen and 2 mm medial to the lateral sacral crest. The angle of the screw is roughly 20° caudal and 30 in the horizontal plane[22-25] (Figs. 12.2A to C). The authors prefer to use fluoroscopy for S2AI screw placement to improve accuracy and maximize screw length. To do this, an AP view is used initially to confirm trajectory cranial to the sciatic notch. Following this, the fluoroscope is rotated 30° cranial for an outlet pelvic view and 30° laterally for an obturator oblique view (roughly in line with the anticipated screw trajectory) to obtain a tear drop view of the inner and outer iliac tables (Fig. 12.3). The goal is to place the screw between the tables on the teardrop view. Using this technique, typically screws around 80 mm in length can be placed with ease and excellent fixation. This technique avoids prominence and the need for connectors as well.

Following obtaining fixation points, attention should be turned to decompression of the spinal canal. This typically requires a laminectomy at least one level above and below the planned osteotomy level. A wide decompression is necessary to avoid impingement of the neurologic elements following osteotomy closure. In the setting of previous decompression, the edge of the previous laminectomy should be established and a sharp cervical curette may be utilized to mobilize scar from the medial aspect of the pedicles and facets. A Penfield dissector can be helpful to mobilize the ventral aspect of the thecal sac in the setting of previous decompression and epidural scarring. Once the central decompression is complete, resection of the superior facet, inferior facet, and pars interarticularis at the osteotomy site should be performed.[2,8,26] Additional partial resection of the inferior facet of the level above and the superior facet of the level below should be performed to gain adequate visualization of the nerve root cephalad and caudal to the pedicle. The transverse processes may then be detached medially from the pedicle at this time and subperiosteal dissection with a Cobb elevator may be performed to adequately expose the lateral wall of the vertebra.

This may be packed with sponges and hemostatic agents to minimize bleeding from segmental vessels that may be encountered in this step.

At this point, the pedicles should be completely free of the surrounding bone. The pedicles and vertebral body should be decancellated with the use of straight and curved curettes. All cancellous bone removed can be saved for bone grafting. Use of hemostatic agents including collagen matrices and thrombin sealants as well as bipolar cautery is critical during this step to avoid excessive bleeding from epidural vessels and cancellous bone. Following decancellation, a Leksell rongeur is used for resecting the pedicles flush with the posterior vertebral body. Care should be taken to retract the thecal sac from the pedicle during this step to avoid nerve root injury.[26]

Following pedicle resection, further decancellation of the vertebral body should be performed utilizing curettes and the high-speed burr as needed. The goal is to thin the posterior vertebral cortex as much as possible. Following this, a reverse-angled curette should be passed between the anterior dura and posterior vertebral cortex and tamped forward to create a greenstick fracture allowing the posterior cortex to be resected symmetrically in accordance with the preoperative plan. At this point, a temporary rod should be placed across the osteotomy site to avoid destabilization.[26]

The authors prefer to use narrow osteotomes at this point to complete the wedge resection of the vertebral body. The goal is to have the osteotome cuts converge at a point on the anterior vertebral cortex to provide a pivot point for the osteotomy.

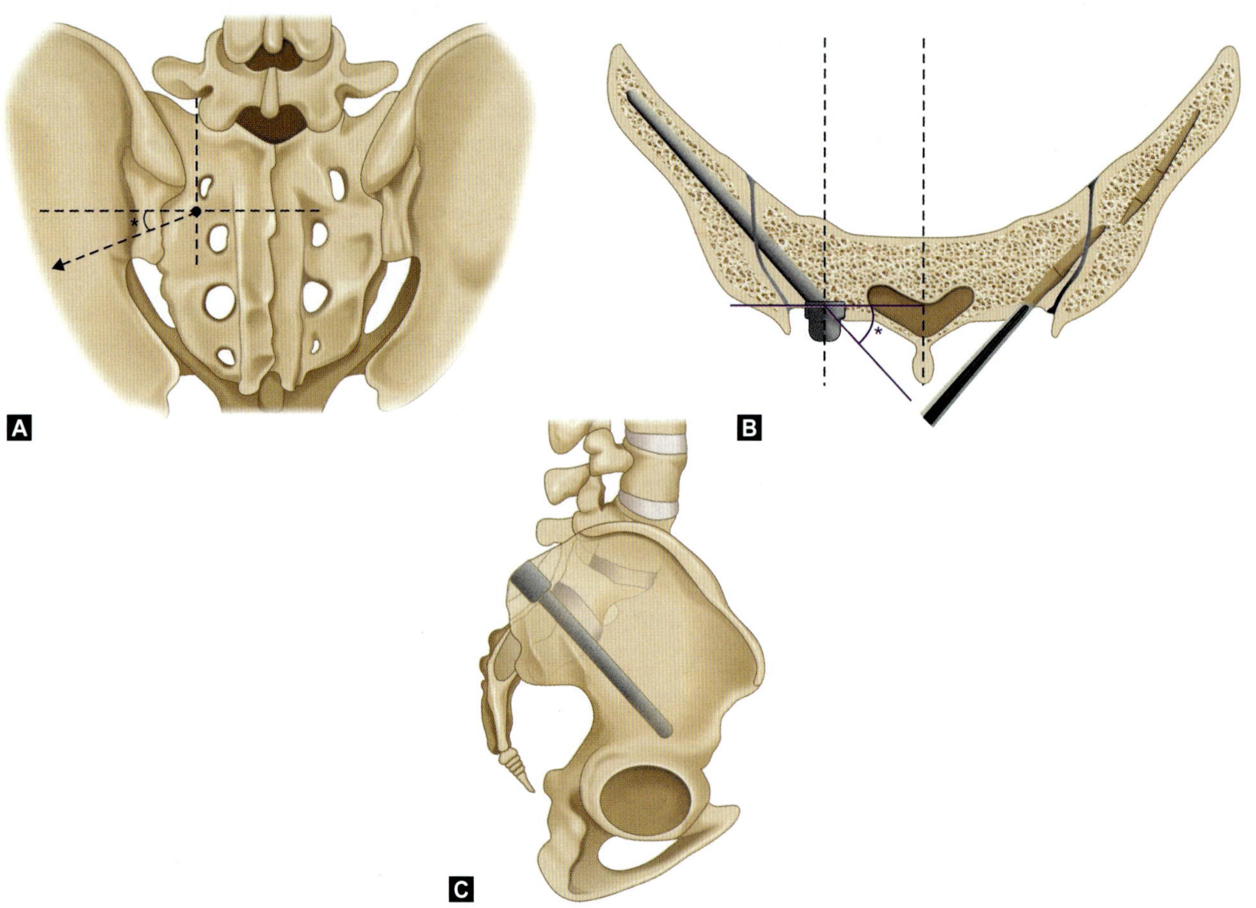

Figs. 12.2A to C: (A) The starting point for S2-alar-ilium screw at the midpoint between the S1 and S2 foramen and 2 cm medial to the lateral sacral crest. (B) Axial view showing the lateral angulation of the gear shift of roughly 30° from the horizon. (C) Lateral view showing the angulation of the screw with a caudal angulation of roughly 20°.
Source: Park JH, Hyun SJ, Kim KJ, et al. J Korean Neurosurg Soc. 2015;58(6):578-81. doi: 10.3340/jkns.2015.58.6.578. Epub 2015 Dec 31. PMID:26819698; HYPERLINK "/pubmed/26819698"

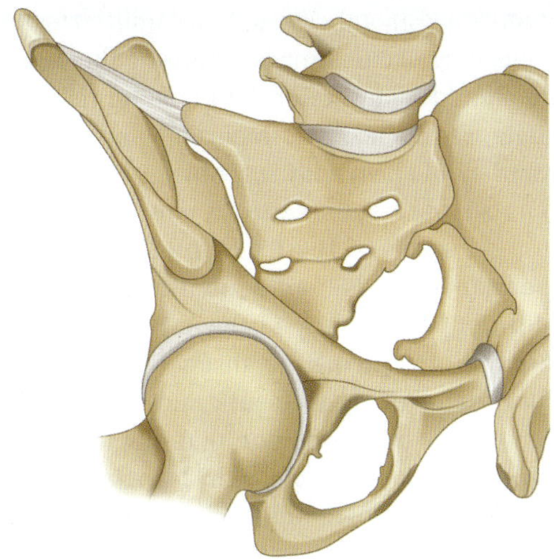

Fig. 12.3: Obturator oblique outlet view, also known as a tear drop view, that should be obtained during fluoroscopically guided cannulation for an S2-alar-ilium screw. Screw path should remain between the inner and outer iliac tables on this view.
Source: El Dafrawy MH, Kebaish KM. Percutaneous S2 Alar iliac fixation for pelvic insufficiency fracture. Orthopedics. 2014;37(11):e1033-5.

Surgeons may choose to use lateral fluoroscopy to assist with this step. The final step in the technique involves resection of the lateral vertebral wall up to the anterior vertebral cortex with a Leksell rongeur to complete the osteotomy on both sides.

Prior to closure of the osteotomy, the authors recommend checking neuromonitoring signals including motor evoked potentials. These should be repeated following osteotomy closure. Before wedge closure, the temporary rod screw connection should be loosened but not removed to serve as a guide for closure. The authors prefer to achieve closure primarily by hyperextending the patient's chest and hips to achieve most of the correction. Compression of the temporary construct is also performed to assist with closure but excessive force, especially in osteoporotic patients, should be used with caution as this can result in instrumentation failure.[2] Care should be taken to avoid fracture of the anterior cortex which may result in subluxation of the osteotomy. Once closure is complete, compression across the lateral bony masses should be ensured to allow for osteotomy healing. In addition, a careful palpation of the thecal sac should be performed with a Woodson elevator to confirm the absence of neural impingment[26] (Figs. 12.4A to C).

Following this, the temporary rod may either be exchanged for a long rod spanning the entire construct or maintained as part of an accessory rod construct. In the absence of prior fusion, the authors prefer to use a dual rod construct which has been shown to provide additional stability at the osteotomy site. Bone grafting and preparation of the remaining fusion bed may proceed in standard fashion. Long radiographs should be obtained if possible to assess final alignment.

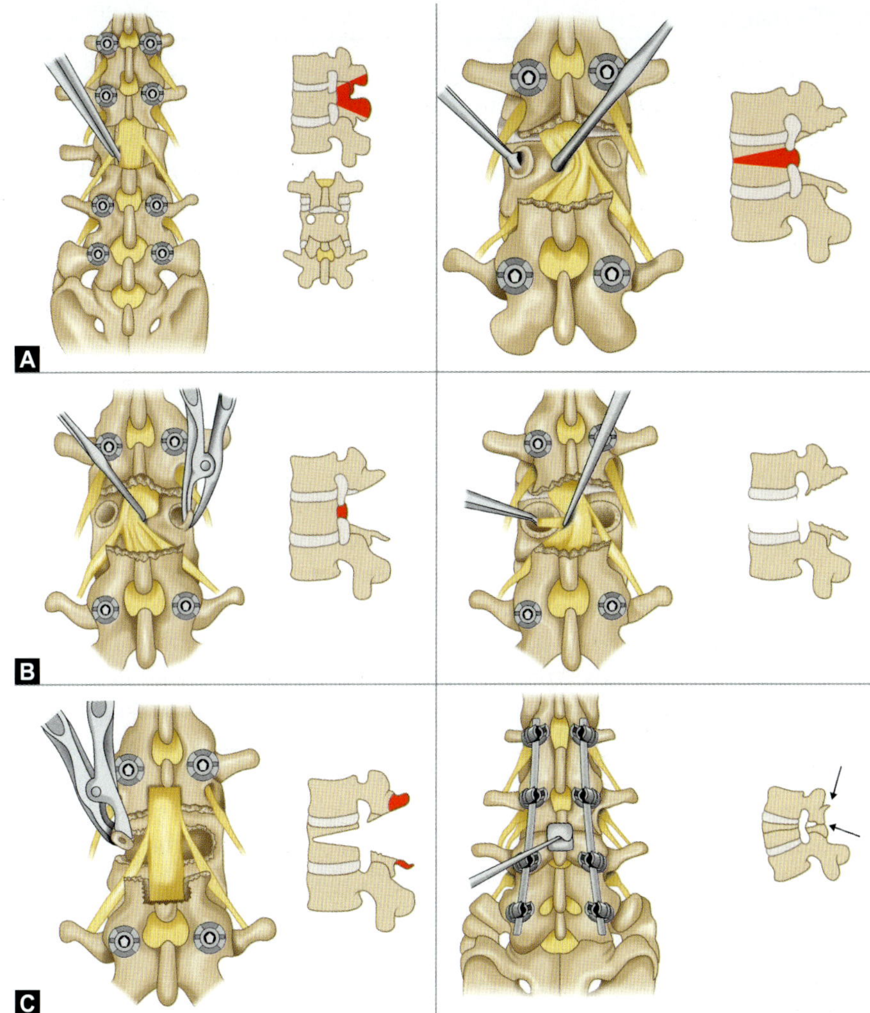

Figs. 12.4A to C: (A) Central laminectomy and facet resection. Decancellation followed by pedicle resection. (B) Resection of the posterior cortex of the vertebral body. (C) Wedge resection of the lateral walls. Closure of the osteotomy and palpation to check for neural impingement.
Source: Bridwell KH, Lewis SJ, Rinella A, et al. Pedicle subtraction osteotomy for the treatment of fixed sagittal imbalance: surgical technique. J Bone Joint Surg Am. 2004;86A:44-50.

Given the prolonged duration and increased blood loss associated with these types of cases, consideration should be given to intensive care postoperatively. The authors use subfascial drains, orthoses, as well as both mechanical and chemical deep vein thrombosis (DVT) prophylaxis as part of the standard postoperative protocol. Patients are mobilized as soon as possible with physical therapy, and standing radiographs are obtained prior to discharge.

OUTCOMES

In a 5-year follow-up study of 35 consecutive patients who underwent lumbar PSO, Kim et al.[27] reported very good patient satisfaction (87%) with good function (69%) and fair pain subscales (66%) at final follow-up. It is important to note that there was no deterioration of outcomes as measured by Oswestry disability index (ODI) and Scoliosis Research Society (SRS) outcome scores from 2 to 5 years. Overall, there were no significant changes in radiographic parameters although many patients did exhibit a gradually increasing SVA with time. Ten pseudarthrosis (29%) occurred in eight patients all of which required revision.[27] However, this did not have any significant effect on long-term outcome scores following revision surgery.

A larger series of 140 patients who underwent PSO with an average of 8-year follow-up supported earlier findings. In this study, the authors found an over 20 point improvement in ODI scores and an over 90% patient satisfaction rate. Average radiographic correction was 36.2° of lordosis.[28]

Experience does seem to play a role in surgical and radiographic outcomes. Choi et al.[29] reported significant reductions in operative time (569.6 vs 392.0 min) and surgical bleeding (1,777.5 vs 949.5 mL) with experience following 40 consecutive PSOs. Furthermore, radiographic correction of SVA and lordosis (25.7° vs 35.8°) were significantly better with experience as well. Not surprisingly, complication rates including intraoperative complications, postoperative neurologic deficits, and revision surgery were lower with greater experience.[29] While these findings caution less experienced surgeons performing these complex procedures, it is important to note that the overall outcome scores did not change with experience.

While pseudarthrosis is a common problem following PSO, revision surgery for this complication can provide good radiographic and clinical outcomes. Kim et al. in a series of 18 consecutive patients undergoing revision for pseudarthrosis after PSO showed significant improvement in SVA and lumbar lordosis following revision.[27,30] Moderate improvements in ODI and SRS outcome scores were observed with a 5-year follow-up. The authors stress the importance of increasing the size and number of implants as well as generous use of bone graft and biologics to achieve a successful result.[30]

COMPLICATIONS

Given the magnitude of this type of procedure, complications occur despite meticulous attention to the surgical technique. Blood loss commonly exceeds 1 L and should be minimized especially during initial decompression and exposure.[2] The authors prefer to use a radiofrequency bipolar hemostatic sealer (Aquamantys™, Medtronic, Minneapolis, MN, United States) which has been validated for reducing blood loss and transfusion rate in multilevel spinal fusion.[31] The authors also routinely used tranexamic acid infusions when not prohibited by patient comorbidities to reduce bleeding as well. Intraoperative blood salvage is also utilized to minimize transfusion requirements. Brisk bleeding occurs especially during the decancellation process. The anesthesia team should be aware of the bleeding risk as well as the risk of coagulopathy. Adequate vascular access is important, and packed red cells, platelets, and fresh frozen plasma should be readily available.

Neurologic deficits are observed frequently postoperatively following a PSO. Buchowski et al. in their series of 108 PSOs found a 11.1% rate of neurologic deficit which was permanent in 2.8% of patients.[32] It is important to note that neuromonitoring did not identify any of these deficits intraoperatively. This highlights the importance of verifying the absence of dorsal compression of the neural elements following osteotomy closure and careful nerve root retraction during pedicle resection. The most common neurologic deficit typically involves transient weakness and radiculopathy related to a single nerve root. Cauda equina syndrome or catastrophic neurologic injury is rare. However, severe neurologic injury can occur if a sudden subluxation occurs during wedge closure. For this reason, surgeons should avoid fracture of the anterior cortex as well as forceful cantilever correction maneuvers.

Surgical site infection is common given the extent of the procedure and the frequency of multiple previous surgeries. Infection rates have been reported to be as high as 7%. These should be treated in standard fashion with surgical debridement and a minimum of 6 weeks of intravenous antibiotics.[2]

Given the degree of correction and long lever arm of most PSO constructs, in addition to pseudarthrosis, patients are susceptible to acute junctional fracture at the proximal end of the construct. In a series of 264 patients who underwent long thoracolumbar fusions, O'Leary et al. identified 13 patients (4.9%) who suffered acute fracture at the proximal end of the construct.[33] This resulted in acute neurologic deficit in two patients and required revision surgery with proximal extension of the fusion in nine patients. Risk factors identified included obesity, older age, and osteopenia.[33] In addition to acute early proximal junctional failure (PJF) with collapse of the proximal segment and subluxation, late failure can occur with adjacent level compression fracture and kyphosis.

Many studies have examined methods to reducing PJF. It is unclear what role the upper instrumented segment plays in failure. According to a study by Kim et al., as long as the upper instrumented vertebra (UIV) includes the neutral and stable vertebra following long thoracolumbar fusion, the exact level is not important regarding risk of PJF, revision, or functional outcomes.[34] Additional options to reduce PJF have been examined including less rigid proximal fixation, supplemental rib fixation, cement augmentation, and dorsal soft tissue preservation.[35,36] However, currently none of these methods offer clear benefits. Regardless, the authors recommend a routine evaluation of bone mineral density and optimization prior to PSO especially in patients with a preexisting diagnosis of osteoporosis or osteopenia.

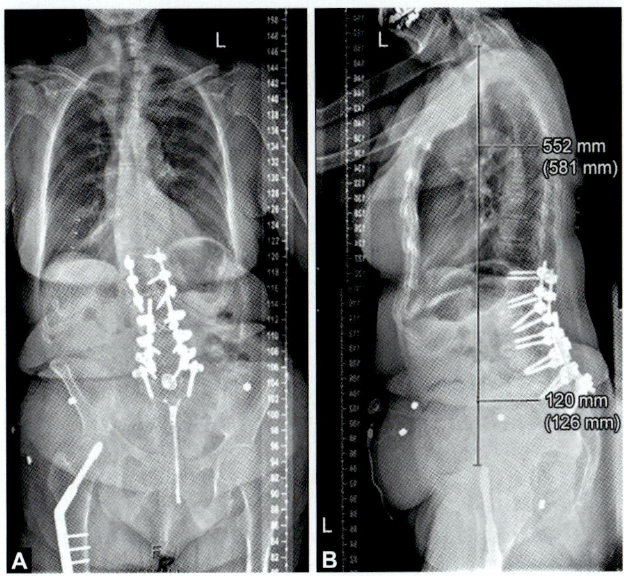

Figs. 12.5A and B: (A) Preoperative anteroposterior radiographs. (B) Preoperative lateral radiograph demonstrating an sagittal vertical axis of 12 cm.

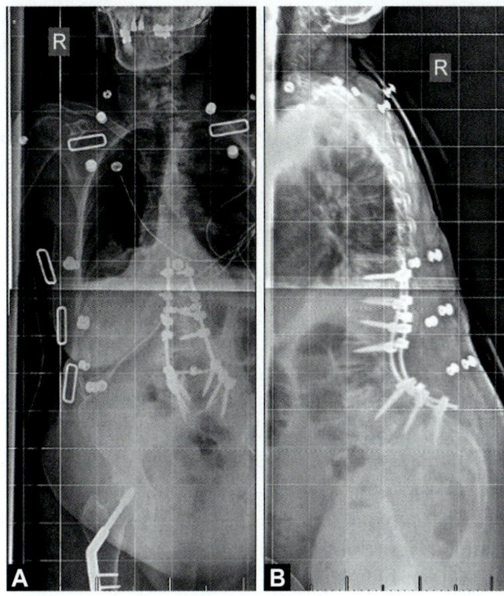

Figs. 12.6A and B: (A) Postoperative anteroposterior radiograph. (B) Postoperative lateral radiograph showing improvement of lumbar lordosis.

CASE PRESENTATION

The patient is a 74-year-old female with a prior history of an L2-S1 decompression and fusion performed over a decade ago. This was followed more recently by a revision T12-L2 decompression and fusion for adjacent segment disease. Following her most recent lumbar surgery, the patient reports progressive lower extremity pain, weakness, and stooped forward posture. She also reported a worsening right-sided truncal shift. These symptoms limit her standing to only 5 min as she develops postural fatigue and back pain. She requires a cane for ambulation which is also significantly limited. Her symptoms have persisted despite comprehensive nonoperative management including physical therapy, epidural injections, nonsteroidal anti-inflammatory drugs (NSAIDs), and opioids.

On physical examination, she is noted to have a right-sided trunk shift and positive sagittal balance. She is unable to extend past neutral in the lumbar spine. She has notable gait instability from a stooped forward posture. A neurologic examination is negative for any signs of myelopathy but does demonstrate some right lower extremity weakness.

An radiographic evaluation demonstrates previous instrumentation from T12-S1 with evidence of fusion mass. There is no evidence of motion in the lumbar spine with flexion and extension images also suggesting a solid fusion. On full length standing radiographs, the patient is noted to have an SVA of 12 cm and a coronal decompensation of 4 cm to the right (Figs. 12.5A and B). The CT scan demonstrates evidence of a possible pseudarthrosis at L2-3 but no evidence of pseudarthrosis elsewhere. An MRI scan shows the previous lumbar decompression and no evidence of recurrent stenosis.

Given the significant sagittal plane deformity and functional disability, the patient was consented to a PSO an L3 with a revision fusion from T10 to S1. Given the solid fusion at L5-S1, it was felt that pelvic instrumentation was not necessary. Since an additional coronal plane deformity was observed, an asymmetric PSO was performed to partially correct the right-sided truncal shift. The operation proceeded without any intraoperative or postoperative complications. Blood loss was estimated at 1,300 mL and the neurologic exam remained stable postoperatively. The patient was discharged to a skilled nursing facility at 7 days postoperatively. At 3 months follow-up, the patient has good correction of both sagittal and coronal plane deformity (Figs. 12.6A and B). She notes minimal lower back discomfort and markedly improved posture and function.

REFERENCES

1. Thomasen E. Vertebral osteotomy for correction of kyphosis in ankylosing spondylitis. Clin Orthop Relat Res. 1985;194:142-52.
2. Wang MY, Berven SH. Lumbar pedicle subtraction osteotomy. Oper Neurosurg. 2007;60:140-6.

3. Bernhardt M, Bridwell KH. Segmental analysis of the sagittal plane alignment of the normal thoracic and lumbar spines and thoracolumbar junction. Spine (Phila. Pa. 1976). 1989;14:717-21.
4. Jackson RP, McManus AC. Radiographic analysis of sagittal plane alignment and balance in standing volunteers and patients with low back pain matched for age, sex, and size. A prospective controlled clinical study. Spine (Phila. Pa. 1976). 1994;19:1611-8.
5. Schwab F, Lafage V, Boyce R, et al. Gravity line analysis in adult volunteers: age-related correlation with spinal parameters, pelvic parameters, and foot position. Spine (Phila. Pa. 1976). 2006;31:E959-67.
6. Lafage V, Schwab F, Patel A, et al. Pelvic tilt and truncal inclination: two key radiographic parameters in the setting of adults with spinal deformity. Spine (Phila. Pa. 1976). 2009;34:E599-606.
7. Bradford DS, Tribus CB. Current concepts and management of patients with fixed decompensated spinal deformity. Clin Orthop Relat Res. 1994;306:64-72.
8. Bridwell KH, Lewis SJ, Lenke LG, et al. Pedicle subtraction osteotomy for the treatment of fixed sagittal imbalance. J Bone Joint Surg Am. 2003;85-A:454-63.
9. Booth KC, Bridwell KH, Lenke LG, et al. Complications and predictive factors for the successful treatment of flatback deformity (fixed sagittal imbalance). Spine (Phila. Pa. 1976). 1999;24:1712-20.
10. Lagrone MO, Bradford DS, Moe JH, et al. Treatment of symptomatic flatback after spinal fusion. J Bone Joint Surg Am. 1988;70:569-80.
11. Legaye J, Duval-Beaupère G, Hecquet J, et al. Pelvic incidence: A fundamental pelvic parameter for three-dimensional regulation of spinal sagittal curves. Eur Spine J. 1998;7:99-103.
12. Brown CW, Orme TJ, Richardson HD. The rate of pseudarthrosis (surgical nonunion) in patients who are smokers and patients who are nonsmokers: a comparison study. Spine (Phila. Pa. 1976). 1986;11:942-3.
13. Schwab F, Ungar B, Blondel B, et al. Scoliosis Research Society. Schwab adult spinal deformity classification: a validation study. Spine (Phila. Pa. 1976). 2012;37:1077-82.
14. Hanson DS, Bridwell KH, Rhee JM, et al. Correlation of pelvic incidence with low- and high-grade isthmic spondylolisthesis. Spine (Phila. Pa. 1976). 2002;27:2026-9.
15. Angevine PD, Bridwell KH. Sagittal imbalance. Neurosurg Clin N Am. 2006;17:353-63, vii.
16. Bridwell KH. Decision making regarding Smith-Petersen vs. pedicle subtraction osteotomy vs. vertebral column resection for spinal deformity. Spine (Phila. Pa. 1976). 2006;31:S171-8.
17. Dorward IG, Lenke LG. Osteotomies in the posterior-only treatment of complex adult spinal deformity: a comparative review. Neurosurg Focus. 2010;28:E4.
18. Kim K-T, Suk K-S, Cho Y-J, et al. Clinical outcome results of pedicle subtraction osteotomy in ankylosing spondylitis with kyphotic deformity. Spine (Phila. Pa. 1976). 2002;27:612-8.
19. Zhao Y, Wang Y, Wang Z, et al. Effect and strategy of 1-stage interrupted 2-level transpedicular wedge osteotomy for correcting severe kyphotic deformities in ankylosing spondylitis. Clin spine Surg. 2017;30:E454-9.
20. Kuhns CA, Bridwell KH, Lenke LG, et al. Thoracolumbar deformity arthrodesis stopping at L5: fate of the L5-S1 disc, minimum 5-year follow-up. Spine (Phila. Pa. 1976). 2007;32:2771-6.
21. Edwards CC 2nd, Bridwell KH, Patel A, et al. Thoracolumbar deformity arthrodesis to L5 in adults: the fate of the L5-S1 disc. Spine (Phila. Pa. 1976). 2003;28:2122-31.
22. Kuklo TR, Bridwell KH, Lewis SJ, et al. Minimum 2-year analysis of sacropelvic fixation and L5-S1 fusion using S1 and iliac screws. Spine (Phila. Pa. 1976). 2001;26:1976-83.
23. Hoernschemeyer DG, Pashuck TD, Pfeiffer FM. Analysis of the S2 alar-iliac screw as compared with the traditional iliac screw: does it increase stability with sacroiliac fixation of the spine? Spine J. 2017;17:875-9.
24. Park JH, Hyun SJ, Kim KJ, et al. Free hand insertion technique of S2 sacral alar-iliac screws for spino-pelvic fixation: technical note, acadaveric study. J Korean Neurosurg Soc. 2015;58(6):578-81.
25. Tsuchiya K, Bridwell KH, Kuklo TR, et al. Minimum 5-year analysis of L5-S1 fusion using sacropelvic fixation (bilateral S1 and iliac screws) for spinal deformity. Spine (Phila. Pa. 1976). 2006;31:303-8.
26. Bridwell KH, Lewis SJ, Rinella A, et al. Pedicle subtraction osteotomy for the treatment of fixed sagittal imbalance. Surgical technique. J Bone Joint Surg Am. 2004;86-A(Suppl 1):44-50.
27. Kim YJ, Bridwell KH, Lenke LG, et al. Results of lumbar pedicle subtraction osteotomies for fixed sagittal imbalance. Spine (Phila. Pa. 1976). 2007;32:2189-97.
28. Kim K-T, Lee S-H, Suk K-S, et al. Outcome of pedicle subtraction osteotomies for fixed sagittal imbalance of multiple etiologies: a retrospective review of 140 patients. Spine (Phila. Pa. 1976). 2012;37:1667-75.
29. Choi HY, Hyun S-J, Kim K-J, et al. Surgical and radiographic outcomes after pedicle subtraction osteotomy according to surgeon's experience. Spine (Phila. Pa. 1976). 2017;42:E795-801.
30. Kim YJ, Bridwell KH, Lenke LG, et al. Pseudarthrosis in adult spinal deformity following multisegmental instrumentation and arthrodesis. J Bone Joint Surg Am. 2006;88:721-8.
31. Frank SM, Wasey JO, Dwyer IM, et al. Radiofrequency bipolar hemostatic sealer reduces blood loss, transfusion requirements, and cost for patients undergoing multilevel spinal fusion surgery: a case control study. J Orthop Surg Res. 2014;9:50.
32. Buchowski JM, Bridwell KH, Lenke LG, et al. Neurologic complications of lumbar pedicle subtraction osteotomy. Spine (Phila. Pa. 1976). 2007;32:2245-52.
33. O'Leary PT, Bridwell KH, Lenke LG, et al. Risk factors and outcomes for catastrophic failures at the top of long pedicle screw constructs a matched cohort analysis performed at a single center. Spine (Phila. Pa. 1976). 2009;34:2134-9.
34. Kim YJ, Bridwell KH, Lenke LG, et al. Is the T9, T11, or L1 the more reliable proximal level after adult lumbar or lumbosacral instrumented fusion to L5 or S1? Spine (Phila. Pa. 1976). 2007;32:2653-61.
35. Nguyen NLM, Kong CY, Hart RA. Proximal junctional kyphosis and failure—diagnosis, prevention, and treatment. Curr Rev Musculoskelet Med. 2016;9(3):299-308.
36. Hyun S-J, Lenke LG, Kim YC, et al. Long-term radiographic outcomes of a central hook-rod construct for osteotomy closure: minimum 5-year follow-up. Spine (Phila. Pa. 1976). 2015;40:E428-32.

Index

Page numbers followed by *f* indicate figures.